Birth Becomes Hers

Choosing Home Birth

Bree Moore

Innate Ink Publishing

BIRTH BECOMES HERS

Copyright ©2019 by Innate Ink Publishing

Second Edition ©2021

Published in the United States of America.

E-books are non-transferable. They cannot be sold, shared, or given away. The unauthorized reproduction or distribution of this copyrighted work is a crime punishable by law. No part of this book may be scanned, uploaded to or downloaded from file sharing sites, or distributed in any other way via the internet or any other means, electronic or print, without the publisher's written permission.

All rights reserved.

Ebook: 978-0-9600087-1-1

Paperback, Second Edition 2021: 978-1-956668-99-5

Hardcover, First Edition 2021: 978-1-956668-01-8

Cover Photography by Utah Birth Stories + Photography

https://www.facebook.com/UtahBirthPhotographer

DISCLAIMER: This book is meant as an educational resource. It is not meant to replace medical advice in the event of an emergency. The author assumes no liability in connection with the use of information contained in this book.

Praise for Birth Becomes Hers

"I couldn't put it down! This book isn't just for those who wish to free birth; it's for every woman who wishes to be empowered toward the birth of her choosing. Bree has put together a wonderful and varied compilation of free birth experiences. Additionally, Birth Becomes Hers offers guidance in the relational aspect of choosing free birth and how it impacts those closest to you. Every woman will be glad they read it!"
   - *Tara L. McGuire author of "Birth Unhindered"*

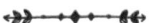

"Reading 'Birth Becomes Hers' is like having a conversation with an extremely knowledgeable and intuitive best friend! Bree's warmth, compassion and understanding come through on every page as she shares her journey from hospital birth to midwife-assisted home birth to freebirth. In addition to Bree's excellent research, she also provides links to articles, podcasts and books that go deeper into the issues many women face when considering having an unassisted birth. Lastly, she allows others to share their own fascinating stories of the challenges and rewards of giving birth at home on their own terms.
   - *Laura Kaplan Shanley, author of "Unassisted Childbirth"*

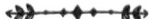

"Bree Moore's faith in life and in the process of childbirth shines like the sun in 'Birth Becomes Hers.' Bree's book is rich in supportive advice, full of inspirational resources and, best of all, packed full with a wealth of diverse freebirth stories! Bree's words ring like the voice of a supportive friend, offering trust in our bodies innate wisdom and strength. I would gladly recommend this book!"

- Sarah M. Haydock, author of "Unhindered Childbirth: Wisdom for the Passage of Unassisted Birth"

Contents

	I
Stories	1
Intuitive Pregnancy and Birth	3
1. Why Choose Freebirth?	4
2. Space and Support	32
3. Getting Your Spouse or Partner On-board	39
4. "Partner Talk" with Tyler Moore	46
5. Self-led Pregnancy	52
6. "Natural" Induction Methods	61
7. Placentas and Post-birth Bleeding	65
8. What if I Tear?	68
9. The Wisdom found in Not-Knowing	73

10. Finding Intuition   77

11. When Fear Comes to Your Birth   81

12. When Birth Ends with Death   90

Freebirth Stories   93

13. The Birth of Juniper Jane Clinger   94

14. Three Days in Labor   105

15. The Power I Always Had: My Home Birth Journey   107

16. The Manifestation of Light & Darkness   110

17. The Freebirth of Oswin Isaac Lund   114

18. 42 Weeks and Counting   118

19. Free to Birth   120

20. 'High Risk' Birth of Rainbow Baby   124

21. Family Birth is the Best Birth   132

22. Birth Works   134

23. An Absolutely Perfect Freebirth   135

24. The Successful Freebirth of Baby J   139

25. The Powerful Birth of Kitty Rose   146

26. A Wild Island Birth   157

27. Accessing Her Inner Power Through Birth	162
VBAC/HBAC Freebirths	171
28. The Birth of Mordekai: Our En Caul Experience	172
29. Freebirth in Autumn	176
30. 3 FBAC of Ansel Finley Dunn	181
31. Anniversary Surprise	184
32. The Breech Birth of Tobie	189
Pleasurable Freebirths	193
33. Birth Before Dinner	194
34. Fast and Pleasurable	198
35. The Truth of the Wild Woman	201
36. Reprogramming My Brain	204
37. Quick and Intense	208
38. Beautiful Harmony and Sweet Surrender	211
39. Fast, Pleasurable Birth of Odena	216
40. First-time Birth, First-time Freebirth	219
41. The Painless Birth of Alexis Will	221
Freebirthing Twins	227

42. The Births of Tristan Karl and Weston Troy	228
Freebirth Miscarriage and Stillbirth	234
43. The Birth of Arrow	235
Freebirth Transfer to Assistance	239
44. A Post-Birth Hospital Transfer	240
45. Intuitive Transfer from Freebirth with Twins	242
More Freebirth Stories	253
46. Ezra's Freebirth	254
47. The Tale of Thea Evelyn	261
48. Birth Like Breath	267
49. Eleven Pounds and Freebirthing	275
50. A Wild Ride	283
51. Tranden Excalibur's Unassisted Birth	293
52. A Christmas Unassisted Birth	299
53. Short and Sweet	305
54. The Freebirth of Eliza May	306
Submit Your Story	316
Resources for Your Birth Journey	317

Read More Birth Stories	320
About the Author	322
Reference	324

To all of my fellow mothers,
past, present, and future.

"There is eternal influence and
power in motherhood."

-Julie B. Beck

Stories

STORIES ARE VITAL TO human existence. From the time man and womankind first began to speak, they communicated through stories.

Stories about the creation of life are one of the most valuable resources available as you prepare to usher your baby earth-side, second only to witnessing birth in person and giving birth yourself.

I value personal, true stories more than studies. Studies provide numbers; cold, hard numbers that may tell the rate or risk of something occurring, but cannot take into account an individual experience, situation, the holistic nature of the body (i.e., that emotions can contribute to physical conditions and circumstances), or the intuition of an expectant woman.

I like studies only because they shut up the naysayers. When birth studies are done well, most often what they reveal is directly in line with what autonomous birthers already know: hands-off, mother-led care is best. Thus, my mantra for those women preparing for birth is this:

Research stories, not studies.

In this book you will find stories. Some of them are mine, most were contributed by others. The stories needed to be told. They needed an outlet into the world. That's all I've done with this book. I've given the stories a place to be told.

This is not a "How-To" book. It is not a book that seeks to answer the question "What is Unassisted birth or Freebirth?" There are several books already available that provide answers and information on these subjects. This book is about experiences. This book is a collection of the knowledge I have gained in the five births I've been privileged to experience personally, and the wisdom found in nearly 40 stories from women around the globe who have come to understand that birth belongs to them.

This book is not meant to convince anyone that freebirth is the only way, the best way, or the right way to give birth. Freebirth is a way. It is a path that one must be summoned to. If you hear the call to give birth free from the medical establishment and unhindered by medical attendants with dubious loyalties or conflicting agendas, then I hope you find inspiration within these pages.

And to those who are not inclined to freebirth, but for whatever reason have found yourself within this book, welcome! May you find some truth or healing to help you on your own journey, either to giving birth yourself or serving women in birth.

Intuitive Pregnancy and Birth

"The knowledge of how to give birth without outside interventions lies deep within each woman."
- *Suzanne Arms*

Why Choose Freebirth?
My Own Journey from Hospital to Home Birth

TO UNDERSTAND WHY I chose freebirth, it would benefit you first to hear my story. I've been blessed to give birth five times, and each one has taught me something new about myself and about birth. From my hospital birth to my third freebirth, they all have intrinsic value. These stories show the journey I have taken. I hope you too find value in these stories, and in the dozens of stories that follow in the second part of this book.

Before freebirth, there was compromise. Before compromise, there was marriage to my husband, Tyler, and getting pregnant 6 months after the honeymoon. Suddenly, it occurred to me that I was going to have a baby, and except for vague recollections from high school health class, I had no idea how to do that. I started reading everything I could find. I discovered the risks of hospital birth and epidurals and immediately decided I would have a natural, unmedicated birth. My husband was hesitant because all of his sisters and his mother had epidurals, so why wouldn't I want one?

We watched "The Business of Being Born" documentary together. He was on board with a natural birth. I convinced him to attend a Hypnobabies childbirth education course with me. He thought it was a bit hokey, but he faithfully attended and supported me. His eyes were opened big-time and he started to really see why I wanted to avoid so many of the interventions that the hospital pushes on mothers during labor.

I saw a group of nurse-midwives during my pregnancy. Everything went textbook perfect. I had labs drawn, did all of the testing, and basically lived in fear constantly that they would find something wrong and that I would have interventions forced on me. But I kept up hope for a natural birth. I did try to talk my husband into having a water birth at home, but being super poor college students at the time, my husband didn't think we had the money for a midwife. He was also very afraid something would go wrong during the labor at home.

So, I compromised. I would have a hospital birth if he would completely support me in having a natural one.

Nearing my due date brought on new fears. My baby was breech. I saw a chiropractor then worried until my baby turned on his own around 36 weeks. I got to 40 weeks and was told I would need to be induced. I said no thanks, so they offered me a non-stress test (NST) the following Monday when I would be just over 41 weeks. I reluctantly agreed, but I knew I didn't want to go to that appointment. I had complete trust in my body and my baby.

I saw a massage therapist friend who agreed to give me an "induction" massage using acupressure. I went into labor 48 hours later, at exactly 41 weeks. My labor started with a big gush of my water all over the kitchen floor. Like kids at Christmas, my husband and I stayed up until 3 a.m. waiting for contractions to start...but they didn't. We called the midwives at the hospital. I was GBS+ and the midwife on-call knew that, but whether she was sleep deprived or just more supportive than I expected, she told us to go to sleep and call in the morning.

I got several hours of sleep and woke up with no contractions, still leaking fluid, and craving bagels. So, naturally, we went to the grocery store. I called my mom, and she wanted to know why I wasn't at the hospital if my water broke. I told her that I didn't want to go in until contractions started. We finished buying my bagels like it was no big deal.

After eating breakfast, I called the midwives again. It was about 10 a.m. at this point. A different midwife was on shift now, one of the ones I really liked because I felt like she was more naturally-minded than the others. Except, when I told her that my water had broken about midnight the night before, she freaked out and said that I needed to come in right away to get antibiotics.

That didn't sit well with me at all. I hung up and told my husband we were waiting a few more hours. I hoped contractions would start before we went to the hospital, but so far there was nothing. We headed into the hospital around 1:30 p.m., not a contraction in sight. They checked me in. A nurse checked me, pushing on my stomach to try and get another gush of fluid, but it never came. She told me my water hadn't really broken, that I was only at 1 cm dilated. I knew she was just being silly because I'd had a massive gush, not just a small one that could have been urine.

She left to call the midwife on-call, and as soon as she left the room there was another enormous gush. When she returned, the bed was dripping and she was pretty shocked. "Oh, I guess your water did break," was kind of the reaction. I felt pretty smug at that. They offered me a hospital gown. I put a tank top on underneath in case I wanted to strip it off during labor. They started an I.V. to deliver antibiotics for GBS, which I agreed to.

I requested intermittent monitoring, which meant they checked baby's heart rate every couple of hours for 15 minutes. They were pretty good about honoring that. The saline-lock in my wrist really bugged me, but I had agreed to the antibiotics and had to have a dose every four hours, so I didn't complain. We walked around the "birth suite" and I bounced on a ball, listening to "Come out, Baby" soundtracks from my hypnosis class.

At 3 p.m. the midwife arrived. She sat me down and talked to me about infections, since my water had been broken for over 12 hours. I felt like a child being lectured to. She mentioned pitocin, and all I could think about was how much I didn't want that. I told her my opinion, and she danced around it, saying it was necessary. I just let it go at that point, saying something complacent to get her to stop talking. She had two women in labor at another hospital, both further along than I was, so she left to tend to them.

Maybe it was all of that Hypnobabies training, or maybe just my personal determination, but I decided I was GOING into labor. My sister came by before anything really happened. She brought food for my husband and chatted for a bit. I remember feeling anxious for her to just leave me alone so I could go into labor. She finally left. During this time my husband was texting his family, giving them updates. I told him to turn off his phone and help me, and to his credit he did. It was finally just us.

The sun was going down, now. As soon as it did, I started feeling contractions, strong and regular. I rocked on my birth ball, on all fours, whatever felt comfortable. My husband was a bit helpless as I dove head-on into labor land. The nurses largely left us alone. I'd had my second round of antibiotics already, and since I wasn't on monitors they didn't have a reason to check on us. At some point the hospital gown came off, and I was just wearing my tank top with no bottoms at all. I ended up pooping around this time. My husband grabbed a towel and cleaned it up. It made us both laugh.

At 5 p.m. a nurse came in with a midwife, someone new. I was so relieved it wasn't the first one! She found me dilated to a 3. No Pitocin for me! I asked her to set me up on the bed with the birth bar. I was squatting and roaring, feeling lots of pressure, but not pushing yet. The midwife expressed concern that I would tire myself out and asked me to get on my back. I agreed, being fully in labor land and just zoned out, very susceptible to suggestion. After all, midwife knows best, right? Once I laid down I knew I wouldn't be getting up.

I hit transition and my peaceful Hypnobirth flew out the window. I was bellowing, I was moaning, I was writhing in bed. I just wanted it to end. I remember praying a lot, feeling like I couldn't do it. My husband held my hand and said comforting things, but felt completely helpless.

I started pushing sometime around 8 p.m. The midwife started coaching me, not counting, but telling me I had to use my energy to push out my bottom instead of yelling. She said if I didn't stop making so much noise she would have me hold my breath. I obeyed, shutting down the urge to make sound, but I kept breathing and she never counted that I recall. They did keep the lights dim, which I'm still grateful for, and it was just the one nurse and the midwife. They had me on my back, holding my legs. To the midwife's credit she did ask if I wanted to move into hands and knees, but by this point I couldn't imagine moving. I said no.

The midwife used olive oil and her fingers to help stretch my vaginal opening, to prevent tearing. She also had a warm compress. I didn't know anything at the time and just let her do it, but it was torture. The ring of fire was intense as it came around his head. This part felt so slow, but in was barely over an hour in full. My son was born with a hand right next to his face, into my husband's waiting hands (we had asked them to let him catch before the birth) by 9:22 p.m., just about 5 hours from the first real contraction.

They clamped the cord almost right away, saying it had stopped pulsing. I know it wasn't done draining when I look back now, but being in the throes of afterbirth exhaustion, I didn't say anything. I was holding my son, admiring him. He pooped on me, which we all laughed about. They asked if they could weigh him, and I said no thanks, that I wanted to hold him longer. They started investigating the tear I'd sustained. It was only a first degree "skid mark" but they insisted on stitching it up a bit. Knowing what I know now, I would have said no to that. Anyway, when they started stitching I handed my son off. My husband crossed the room with him while he was weighed at 8 lbs, 12 oz! So big! And I had done it without medication. I was so relieved at that.

I looked at my husband the next day and told him the next baby would be born at home. He laughed.

My son and I struggled with breastfeeding the first three months due to a painful thrush infection in my breasts from the rounds of antibiotics. Otherwise, our postpartum time and that first year was filled with all the joy and discoveries of first time parents. We co-slept for the first 6 months after attempting to use a crib, and then he started crawling off the bed. We kept him in our room until he was 9 months old and it just felt right to put him in his own space. It was difficult at times, but we were so blessed with good health and plenty of support from family and friends. I almost couldn't wait until we had another.

11 months later, I was the one laughing when I showed my husband the positive pregnancy test. I went dutifully to my first few prenatals with the midwives from my last pregnancy, thinking I had to have some care (I still had such a long way to go). I received an ultrasound that told us we were having a girl, then I said goodbye and transferred to an unlicensed midwife in my area. Traditional or unlicensed midwives are legal in the state of Utah. I didn't realize at the time how lucky I was to have that so readily available.

That midwife was a gem in my eyes. I was able to refuse GBS and Glucose testing. Since I was GBS positive last time she helped me use probiotics preventatively. She lent us a tub for our planned water birth. I dug into visualizing a peaceful water birth at home, using a vision board and fear-clearing throughout my pregnancy. I dabbled with my hypnosis tracks, but didn't feel like it had done much for me in my first labor and didn't plan to use it this time around.

My husband had more confidence in my ability to give birth, but still had financial concerns. We're religious folks, so we prayed about it and decided to move forward with hiring the midwife, having faith that the means would be available. And they were. We happened to find an incredibly supportive midwife with the lowest fee rate in the area, and she let us pay using an affordable monthly plan. Somehow the money was there to pay her every month, despite my husband still being in school and me not working. God truly moves in mysterious ways.

Again, my baby was breech as I neared my due date. My midwife was willing to deliver breech, but preferred not to. She had me using a tilt board to get baby disengaged so she would have room to move. I used flashlights, frozen bags of peas, and chiropractic adjustments, along with visualization, until my baby moved head-down.

I was feeling large and impatient. I thought for sure she would come early, but when the due date (April 25th) came and went, we were still waiting. Friends and family comforted us with words of encouragement, a few meals, and help with my first child. I felt HUGELY pregnant, very uncomfortable at night and tired during the day, but otherwise healthy and happy. I love being pregnant, and despite how difficult it is to wait, I am blessed with immense health and joy in carrying my babies inside me.

I was starting to wonder how big this little girl would be, however, when I weighed in at 182 lbs at my 41 week appointment. I weighed 8 lbs more than I had with my first! I kept trying to assure myself I just had more water, or a bigger placenta, but I was worried she was going to be enormous! I asked my massage friend for another induction massage. She complied, and again, within 48 hours I went into labor. I was exactly 41 weeks.

On Friday, May 3rd, I woke up to a peaceful sunny morning and a small—very small—rush of fluid. I went to the bathroom and emptied my bladder, then laid down again, trying to decide if my water had broken. No more gushes came, so I went about my morning as usual, warning my husband that it MIGHT have been my water and texting the midwife. Tyler and I went shopping, hoping the walking might jumpstart labor. We bought him a new suit at the mall, went home for lunch and naps, and then went back out to a clothing tent sale where I bought some new shirts. I suspected that IF my water had broken, labor would wait until the sun went down, and I was right! It was after dinner, around 7:30 p.m..

Tyler was putting Sam to bed, and I had a contraction that made me stop and think for a moment. I grabbed a pen and started timing. For the next hour I sat there, feeling waves coming at 5-8 minute intervals. I could talk through them, and walk through them, but I still texted the midwife. She was heading back from Salt Lake and I asked her to come by and check me for dilation. She arrived at 9:45 p.m. and we found out I was dilated to 5 centimeters—halfway, baby! She left to meet up with her assistant and grab the rest of her supplies.

We called my Doula and birth photographer and started filling the tub. It felt heavenly! I loved laboring in the water. My biggest regret from this birth is that we sent my son, 18 months old at the time, to be watched by my sister. He was sleeping, and I really just wish we had kept him home through the birth. He had a hard time adjusting because my sister kept him for two days after the birth, so he came home and there was a little intruder in mommy's arms! It caused so many struggles in the year after my daughter was born.

The tub felt great, and I think I needed it to have my own space with so many people crowded in our little apartment, but I hated being in the water and not having full mobility. In retrospect I realize I was trying to have the "perfect" home birth, with a Doula and photographer and everything else. I didn't really need any of it, and being watched definitely contributed to what happened next.

My midwife arrived sometime around 11 p.m. Time was hazy to me now, and all that mattered was the rest I got between contractions. The midwife checked me again (although I can't remember if she checked me in the water or out), and I was at 7 centimeters. Good progress! She asked if we would like to say a prayer, which is something she does during every birth she attends. We said yes, and my husband decided to say it. All I remember about the prayer (I went through a contraction during it) was that he prayed that I would recognize the angels that surrounded me in that time, that they were beings I was familiar with. It was a beautiful prayer, and I felt so blessed by it.

Emotionally, I was ready to have this baby. Physically, I still had a little ways to go. I began telling myself to open, open, OPEN. I would chant it to myself during waves of pressure, which were beginning to become overwhelming and painful. I told everyone I was opening and big as the world. I began to tell myself I couldn't do this. I couldn't go through another contraction. I needed my baby out NOW. I began to bargain…three more contractions, and then you're out, baby. The third one would pass and a fourth one come on and I started voicing all of my doubts out loud to my birth team. They responded with so much love and support. I can't do this, I would say. You ARE doing it, they would reply.

At one point I remember asking "how will I know she's coming?" Thinking about it now is a little funny because it was kind of obvious that she was on her way! I think what I meant was, how much longer do I have to do this? I wanted someone to say something like, "Only ten more minutes," because then it would be more bearable, knowing there was a definitive end. But no one did. They just assured me she was coming, that she would be here soon, that I could do this. I recognized at one point that I was in transition, and that meant she was really close to coming, because transition comes right before full dilation and pushing.

I no longer knew, or cared, what time it was. My husband was in the water with me at this point, and I alternated between crouching, leaning on the side of the tub, and relaxing back against him. The waves of pressure overwhelmed me, and I began grunting and moaning, trying everything I could to relieve the pressure bearing down on me. Being able to move around so easily in the water saved my sanity—if I had been on land, moving would have felt impossible.

I'll say this about labor pain. First, it is impossible to express in the English language how it really feels to give birth. The only word we have is pain, but that word, by itself, is inadequate. This isn't the kind of pain someone feels when they break a bone, or when you stub your toe, or when you get a cut. This is the kind of pain that is an intense workout, which is filled with pressure and the burn of your muscles under that pressure, and as soon as you stop the workout the pressure and apparent pain melt away and you feel so much relief you could sleep. It's true that I practically dozed off between contractions, resting and breathing and feeling immense relief that I never had to experience that contraction again. I also felt immense satisfaction, knowing my baby was that much closer to being born.

It was around this time my midwife suggested that we break my bag of waters, or amniotic sack. It had never fully broken since that tiny gush Friday morning, so it was still intact. The midwife felt that I would feel some relief from my water being broken. She said she had to do it during a contraction, which I wasn't sure I could handle. While she was waiting for my answer a contraction came on and I essentially said, "Here's one now if you're going to do it..." she said she wasn't going to do it during that one, and I felt my body bear down and then a POP! like a water balloon had burst inside of me, and a huge rush of fluid poured out of my body into the water of the birth tub.

I gasped, "That was my water! It just broke!" And everyone kind of laughed and cheered. The midwife said she should have suggested it sooner, making us laugh again. Unfortunately, I didn't notice any change in pressure, probably because baby was coming down so fast and I was still trying to push her out as quickly as possible. I wanted her HEREand NOW. I don't know how long I pushed after my water broke. Maybe half an hour? It didn't feel very long. But in the moment it felt like forever. (I just asked my midwife how long it was —she said my baby was born 34 minutes after my water breaking).

I began to despair that she was going to take several more hours to come, and I didn't feel like I could do that. I prayed and asked for my maternal ancestors to be with me.

It was also at this time that I had to feel my progress. I NEEDED to know my baby was close. I reached down and inside myself. My midwife asked if I could feel her head. I could! It was soft and VERY wrinkly, because her head was being compressed as it molded through my body. The best part, which I announced with a cry of surprise, is that she had hair, and I could feel it! After a few more contractions I asked if Tyler wanted to feel her head and he said yes, and it didn't feel strange at all for him to also reach inside me and touch her head. He says it was incredible to have that experience.

Knowing she was so close motivated me like crazy. Richelle (my midwife) had to keep reminding me to let go of trying to be in control and let my body do what it needed to do, to open slowly and let her descend so there would be little tearing. I was in such a primal state of mind this was really difficult to do. Although I tried, I could hardly prevent what happened next. I began to feel her head start to crown, the slight burning of the ring of fire as her head approached the opening of my body. Each push would bring her almost to the point of coming out, and each time I relaxed her head would retreat back inside of me.

Feeling her so close, and feeling that acute, burning pain, I decided she was coming out. I was roaring at this point, literally letting out a deep, guttural roar with each push. No one attempted to silence me or tell me what to do. I touched her head, felt her crown during one contraction, felt her head almost come out, and decided to keep pushing after the contraction let off.

A few seconds more of burning and then her head was out. I told everyone, who seemed to react with disbelief. My husband says he looked down and saw her head and it was pretty surreal. He reached down, still in the water with me, ready to catch her. The next contraction came and I roared as her shoulders (more burning and pain this time) and the rest of her body was thrust from my body. I was panting from exertion, and my head was ringing a little from the memory of the burning pain I felt at pushing her out.

I can remember everyone seeming to scramble a little, the midwife giving my husband instructions to pass the baby to me, as she couldn't reach the baby from where she was. Tyler passed the baby between my legs and I pulled her up out of the water. The cord was draped over, but not around, her neck, so we slid it off and I sat back against Tyler's chest and put the baby against my chest. The world stopped for a moment. She didn't cry, just looked around for a moment at all of us, adjusting, and then she let out a wail. Tyler looked between her legs, double checking that she was, in fact, a girl. He announced it, and then I had to check too to be sure.

I started to cry a little bit, so relieved that it was over at last, and hardly able to believe that the pain and pressure were gone. We sat in the tub for a while, and then everyone helped us get out of the tub and we headed over the couch after toweling off. I sat on the couch (which was covered, of course) while we waited for the placenta to come. I had a few more mild contractions, nothing very painful, just uncomfortable. Our baby girl's umbilical cord was still intact, and I was holding her and we were covered with a towel on top. Labor was a speedy 6 hours total.

My placenta came out without any cord traction or management, just a few pushes. Everyone exclaimed how big and healthy it was (turns out it was about twice the size of the average placenta… wow!). The cord wasn't cut and clamped until over an hour after the birth. At that point my midwife had gone to another birth that was happening at the same time as mine (crazy how that happens!), and her assistant helped us clean up and get settled. It was about 5 a.m. when we were finally alone with the baby. She hadn't been weighed yet because the midwife had taken the scale, and we hadn't quite chosen a name. In the quiet hours of the morning, before we fell asleep, we decided what she would be called.

Zerushadai, taken from the Hebrew name (found in Numbers 1:6) of Zurishaddai, which means "Rock of the Almighty." We call her Rusha.

When the midwife returned the next day around 11 a.m., we weighed our baby. She was 9 lbs 2 oz, bigger even than her brother had been! But she measured shorter than him at 20 inches even. What a chunky beautiful baby girl she was! And I felt every extra ounce, I'll tell you.

I found out I tore a bad 2nd degree. Getting that stitched up was the worst experience EVER. We were able to have the midwife do it at home, fortunately. That was my worst recovery. I still wonder sometimes what would have happened if I didn't get stitched up. I never saw the extent of the tear, I just wonder.

A mere eight months later we got another pink line. It was earlier than I wanted. I had to supplement my daughter because my milk dries up with pregnancy and I couldn't find donor milk, and that was really difficult for me emotionally. I wanted to breastfeed my daughter, who was still very young, but there just wasn't any milk.

Around this time I took a training to become a Doula. This training was unique. They offered "experiential exercises" to help us understand pelvic anatomy by giving each other pelvic exams. It's the reason I felt drawn to this training; it seemed so different from the sterile nature of the others, like DONA. The workshop was by the company ToLabor. I don't know if they still do the exercises or not. At the time, opting into these experiences was completely optional. The pelvic exam was first. It was handled with complete respect. They covered all the windows and locked the door of our classroom, after those who didn't want to participate left.

You had to agree to allow someone to do a pelvic exam on you in order to practice it yourself. I was pregnant, so I was automatically unable to participate for safety reasons, but one of the women there offered to go through it twice so I could participate. It was a surreal experience, respectfully handled and there was so much love in that room as we all discovered the wonder of the female body and how every part relates to giving birth.

For the second experience they invited a group of pregnant women in to allow us to palpate their bellies and listen with a fetoscope. They emphasized this was "out of scope" for a Doula, but wanted us to understand the parts of pregnancy and birth in a deeper way. These experiences started me on my unassisted birth path before I even started considering it. I never certified as a Doula, just started attending births, a few here and there during that pregnancy.

We had moved, so I started looking for another home birth midwife. Interviewed a couple, picked one, had our first prenatal at 14 weeks. We couldn't find the heart rate with her Doppler, so she told us to get an ultrasound, so I did. Ultrasound showed a healthy baby boy.

The second prenatal was worse. The midwife started telling me she wanted to order all this lab work and talked about the testing she did. If my baby happened to be breech we would have to transfer, if I went over 42 weeks we would have to transfer. I didn't like that. I told her I would refuse most, if not all the testing. She asked me why I wanted a midwife, then. She told me that I would endanger her reputation with the hospital if we ended up transferring and she didn't have those test results. As much as I could see her point, I was completely turned off by her fear. She actually suggested I look into unassisted birth.

I looked into it and never looked back. I told my husband I wanted an unassisted birth, and he was very opposed to the idea. He'd come a long way to accepting home birth, but not having a midwife there was a big trip for him. He asked what would happen if I died, or started bleeding, if baby was breech, etc. I'm a big researcher. I started pulling up studies about the likelihood of those things happened and asked him to read them. Being my partner in all things, he did, and he gradually came around. I fired my midwife and we started doing my own prenatal care.

I read Laura Shanley's "Unassisted Childbirth" book and everything I could find online. We went the whole nine yards: blood pressure, bought our own doppler, weight checks. I think I was trying to mimic mainstream prenatal care so my husband would be more at ease. I know better now!

We didn't tell anyone our plans. I wanted to see it through, first. Most family and friends knew we had a home birth with a midwife before, so when they asked about this time I just said we were having a home birth. In the beginning, I had given them the name of the midwife I planned to hire. Later on I just didn't share that our plans had changed.

I was in my third trimester when I went to visit my parents in Virginia. I felt like sharing, so I told them about our plans to birth unassisted. They had lots of questions. They mostly wanted to make sure that I wasn't going without a midwife because we couldn't afford it, and offered to pay for one. I declined, saying that having an unassisted birth felt right. My parents were respectful and didn't try to pressure me into anything. They just asked about my plans in case there was an emergency, and left it at that.

I was truly tested with this baby! She waited long after her siblings did to be born. I still wonder if her estimated due date was off, since I never had a period between her and her sister. As 42 weeks passed my mother in law asked when "they" would be inducing me. I said "they" wouldn't and that we would keep checking on the baby, and as long as everything was well we would still birth at home.

We lived next door to her, in the basement of her mother's house, and she didn't know our plans to have an unassisted birth. My husband's grandmother didn't either, though she was supportive of us giving birth in her home with a midwife. "That's how I was born," she said, laughing. This incredible woman had nine kids. Her mother had eleven, including a set of twins and a set of triplets all born at home. I was so grateful that she supported my plans to birth at home.

My oldest son (almost 3) had a fever on the 13th of September. My husband cancelled his appointments for the next day, just feeling he needed to stay home. He was starting to get anxious to let the pregnancy go much longer, so we did our own little "stress test" at home by checking my blood pressure and checking baby's heart rate with a Doppler. Baby's kicks were strong and we felt confident waiting a few more days, at least.

We had been having sex regularly several times a week even at this point, which just goes to show that babies come when they are ready. I wanted to avoid all other induction methods, however natural. This time there would be no induction massages, just trust in my body, my baby, and birth.

Anyway, early the next morning at 42 weeks + 3 days, I felt twingy and cranky. About 10 a.m. I couldn't handle having the kids around. We put my daughter down for a nap and sent my son to my mother in law's house next door. We started a card game to pass time. We flirted and really felt some chemistry. I'd wanted to try having sex in labor, so we messed around a bit until we heard my husband's older brother upstairs visiting with Grandma. Awkward! We snuggled and kissed some more, then I started feeling kind of nauseated so we got dressed and went back to the card game.

I started breathing hard through contractions. I didn't want a water birth this time, but I did have a friend who was going to support me during this birth, more for my husband's peace of mind than anything. I called her and asked her to stay upstairs for a while. She did our dishes and made me a bagel.

Contractions were strengthening now. Desperation and a strong longing to be done with labor filled me. I started voicing my fears. I told Tyler I didn't want to have this baby anymore. A bit late for that! My husband was an incredible comfort during this time, which we soon recognized was transition.

I had taught my husband counterpressure and Rebozo during this pregnancy, and he used both to help me cope. I find his touch very relaxing when I'm in labor. I had beautiful Celtic music playing. My husband was using the Rebozo on my behind while I rested on all fours, "shaking the apple tree" or "motorcycle" is what the move is called. It felt SO GOOD. Labor was really intense. I kind of worried about grandma hearing me and felt my space invaded a bit by that. Luckily, my husband's brother had gone home by now.

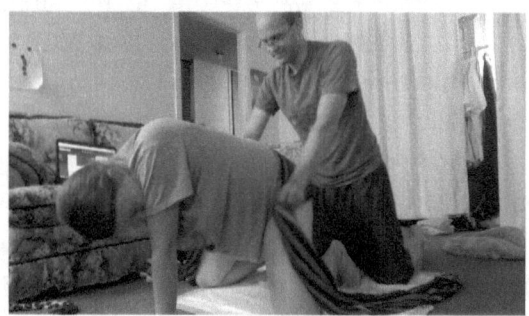

I invited my Doula downstairs to help us. She got me coconut water and took a few pictures since my husband was the one massaging and giving me counterpressure. I used mantras like "easy" to get through transition, checked myself and felt the water sac bulging. Breaking my water felt intuitive. I gave the bag of waters a pinch during a contraction and it burst right away. The pressure increased INSANELY. I slowed things down, though, visualizing my baby sliding out of me.

At one point I felt a cervical lip in place, kind of holding baby up. Following my intuition and my body's cues, I used my fingers to pull the cervical lip aside. It was a VERY intense sensation, but it didn't hurt at all because I could feel how hard to pull to get it out of the way. At that point, I knew I was complete and kept my hand inside me to feel my baby come down the birth canal. COOLEST FEELING EVER. That really helped me control my pushing so I didn't tear.

Baby crowned with a major ring of fire just like my other ones, and then the head was out.

My husband mentioned there was a cord around her neck and quietly slipped it off. He knew just what to do in the moment! The rest of her slid out into his hands, all 9 lbs 7 oz of her! She was HUGE to me. And yes, I said HER. The ultrasound was wrong (surprise) and our baby boy was actually a girl. She was born after nine hours of labor, sweet and slow, my longest but easiest labor so far.

Her placenta was stickier than my first two, taking almost two hours to come. Afterbirth contractions were so painful I was convinced I was having another baby until the placenta came out, fully intact and without excessive bleeding. I used a mirror the next day to check for tearing and to my absolute shock and thrill found NONE. My biggest baby and no tearing! I finally had a nice, easy recovery with no stitches.

Took us three days to name our sweet surprise girl. Then, at about three weeks old she got a viral infection, most likely from a visiting relative, and ended up in the hospital. I stayed with her the entire time. She contracted spinal meningitis and was life-flighted to Primary Children's Hospital, but I never felt panicked. I just felt calm. I believe her coming "late" helped her to fight the illness and cope with the medical treatment she was subjected to. I advocated for her, refusing care I believed was unnecessary. They pumped her full of antibiotics, unfortunately, afraid that it was a bacterial infection. The results came back on day five that it was viral and I pushed for them to let us go home that day. They did, luckily.

There was never any flack from my husband's mother or grandmother about the unassisted birth. My mother-in-law was shocked, but I think just relieved everything went well.

I got pregnant next with baby #4 when our 3rd was 12 months old. At this point we have kids aged 4, 2, and 1. Life is busy, but we want a lot of kids, so it all just felt very natural to not prevent pregnancies. I'm glad I had more space between these two, though. We planned for another unassisted birth and pregnancy. I was very low maintenance and hardly did any prenatal checks, just made sure I was healthy and that I felt good. I think we checked my blood pressure a couple times and listened with a fetoscope. It felt normal by now. My husband is a big proponent for home birth and very proud of our ability to do it ourselves, he tells everyone he meets!

We've both come a long way.

My pregnancy was uneventful. We did have an ultrasound. It's one thing we appreciate having, to make sure that there are no serious defects. We're aware of the risks, but the pros outweigh the cons for us and it doubles as the proof of pregnancy we need for a birth certificate. A local freestanding birth center provides them at a pretty decent rate.

So we found out it was another girl, our 3rd. I'd been hoping for another boy, but we love babies and moved past any disappointment quickly. We ended up moving to our own home, which was nice. I hired a Doula again, mostly to help with our other three children in case I gave birth during the day. She has training as a shamanic healer and helped me work through some fears, especially as my due month came up. I didn't want to go late with this one. I wasn't sure I could last as long as I did with my third. I joked with my husband that if we had a baby smaller than 9 lbs she would shoot right out of me…be careful what you wish for!

The night of her estimated due date, I was putting together a birth playlist. I started to feel something around 9 p.m. I thought they were practice contractions. I decided to take a shower, and they got more intense. Told my husband we should go to bed in case this was the real deal. We never made it.

We did get to have sex, though! I told my husband it was his last chance for several weeks and he took me up on the offer. It wasn't a remarkable experience for me, but I enjoyed the connection and intimacy, and it did speed things up. Things got intense REALLY fast after that.

We called our Doula but told her it wasn't quite time for her to come. My husband mostly ran around gathering our supplies. I'm very vocal during transition. I typically start saying I can't do it, it's taking too long, etc. My husband says he was laughing inside every time I said that because this labor was moving FAST. I recognized I was in transition, but the conscious and logical side of my brain was afraid I'd be in transition for hours.

My water broke. I was on all fours on top of our bed. I checked myself and I was complete. I'm pushing. My husband called our Doula, bless his heart. She lived just 10 minutes away.

Remember how I said be careful what you wish for? This baby FLEW around my pubic bone. Massive fetal ejection reflex (FER). I started panting as she crowned, telling her to slow down. Her head came out. I thought it was a butt until I felt her nose. She shot out in the next contraction.

I couldn't believe how fast it happened! My Doula came in a few moments later, just 20 minutes after we called her.

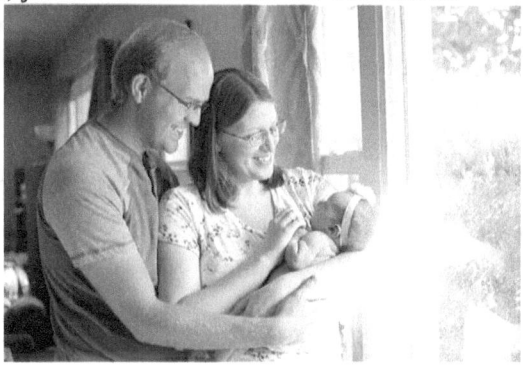

Total birth time was about four hours. This placenta stuck again, but came after about two hours as I squatted over a bowl after cutting our baby's cord. Again, there was no tearing, despite how fast her head came out. Recovery was easier.

I did develop postpartum anxiety a few months after her birth. Four little ones at home and running two small businesses is no joke! I balanced my hormones with Seed Cycling and diet and the anxiety disappeared. I worked slowly towards losing the bit of extra weight I gained during my pregnancy.

I'm a trained postpartum belly binder. I've used it after four of my five births, and it's dramatically helped my healing. I teach workshops locally and have online courses for birth professionals and also women wanting to do it themselves at www.learnbellybinding.com.

My 5th pregnancy was uneventful. Rather boring, truth be told! By now everyone who knows me knew my preference for unassisted pregnancy and birth, and I'm fortunate to also have their respect. Aside from asking how I was feeling and how the pregnancy was going every so often, my family and friends didn't have much to say.

At five weeks I told my husband. At about 14 weeks we started telling everyone else. At 22 weeks we had an ultrasound that told us we were finally having another boy. Our kids were thrilled!

One of the biggest stressors for me was my hip and lower back pain. I tried everything I could think of and afford, from energy healing to massage to chiropractic. The only thing that helped was NOT exercising. I prayed I wouldn't get too unfit, as I couldn't even take short walks.

We were preparing to move most of my pregnancy in order to be closer to my husband's new job, so there was quite a bit of apprehension about where I would be giving birth. I kept an emergency birth essentials bag packed so we would be ready to have this baby no matter where we were in the moving process. We ended up in our new home the weekend before Christmas. With renovations to do on the floors there was a lot of stress, but we managed to get through it.

Around 34 weeks I had started to wonder if our baby would come early. Braxton Hicks contractions started around this time too. We thought it might be fun to have a Christmas or New Year's baby, but he had other plans. We continued praying and kept our faith for a healthy pregnancy and birth.

The estimated due date we tracked this pregnancy by was January 19th. It came and went. I was so uncomfortable and emotional. I wanted this baby to come! I got a chiropractic adjustment and a massage that week, and felt good about accepting an additional acupressure "induction massage" during it. I told my baby that I wasn't trying to force him, but if he was ready, then now was a great time to come. This was all part of me trying to make sure my body was completely ready to give birth.

Two days later, the morning of January 25th, I woke up knowing something was different. Starting at 7 a.m., I felt regular contractions about every eight minutes. I kissed my husband and sent him off to work without telling him, knowing this could still be a false alarm. He left and I rested in bed, watching the minutes pass and trying not to get too excited. The older kids woke up, and I got them breakfast. The contractions petered out, probably from all the noise and distraction, and then started up again when the kids went downstairs to play. I started calling babysitters.

The contractions were still 8 minutes apart, but getting stronger. I breathed through them and started getting things ready, mostly trying to ready my mind. For some reason, despite having done this four times before and despite all of my mental preparation, I felt so nervous about coping through the pain! I think my subconscious knew that this birth would be difficult.

We planned on my husband's mother helping with the kids, since she lives down the street from our new home, but she wasn't available right away. Instead, I felt impressed to call a dear friend of mine who lives an hour away. She was prepared to leave immediately, despite me never having asked her previously if she would watch our kids during the birth.

The next call was to my husband. He's a math teacher at a junior high school, so I called the front office. They thought I was a student and transferred my call to the counselor's office, haha! Fortunately, they figured out who I was and what I needed and promised to call my husband right away. He arrived home about twenty minutes later. The cramping was hard by this point, though still five minutes apart. I tried to find a rhythm. My husband's questions were getting annoying.

I called the birth photographer. I still didn't know if I wanted her there, but she lived an hour north and I wanted to give her time to get here. When she finally arrived, I signed some paperwork I hadn't gotten a chance to during pregnancy, and then I asked her to wait in her car until I was ready. I could still sort of talk through contractions at this point. I decided to labor in the master bedroom after that. It was cozy and felt intimate. Brightly lit by daylight, which was added to by the warm glow of a salt lamp. I turned on my

"Greatest Showman" station on Pandora. It was great music to dance and sing to as contractions became more serious, longer and closer together.

Then, things got messy. My word for this labor is "gritty." It was hard, it was a bit gross, it was exceptionally painful. At this point I just wanted the baby out. I didn't want to have to do contractions anymore, didn't want to face the pain. I felt a strong desire to break my water, but part of me knew it was too soon. I wanted my water to break so that I knew I was closer to being done. I prayed and asked inside myself, When I should break my water? The answer I received was, Wait at least three contractions. Three. I can do three.

I went to the bathroom, deciding to labor on the toilet for a while and feeling the urge to poop. TMI, but my stool was very soft. Contractions in the bathroom were hard, but I also appreciated how natural it felt to sit on the toilet in labor. Something about it helped me open up a bit, at least energetically if not literally.

I impatiently waited the three contractions, my hand inside my vagina the entire time, feeling the hard mass that I knew was my baby's head. It felt so far away! Each contraction made the amniotic sac bulge like a balloon. During the fourth contraction, I gripped it between my thumb and forefinger and pinched hard. My fingers slipped at first, and then it popped, water gushing into the toilet. I yelled to my husband that my water broke. He told me he knew, that he had heard it, and brought me a towel so I could walk to the bedroom. It took me a minute, as contractions got stronger after my water broke.

I don't have words to describe what the contractions felt like. Pain seems inadequate. I wondered what an epidural might feel like. I didn't want one, but I did want the pain to end. I labored on my hands and knees on my bedroom floor, towels and chux pads between me and the carpet. My husband texted the birth photographer after I told him to invite her in. I could always ask her to leave if I didn't want her there. She slipped into the room and got into our closet, which was in front of me, and started taking pictures.

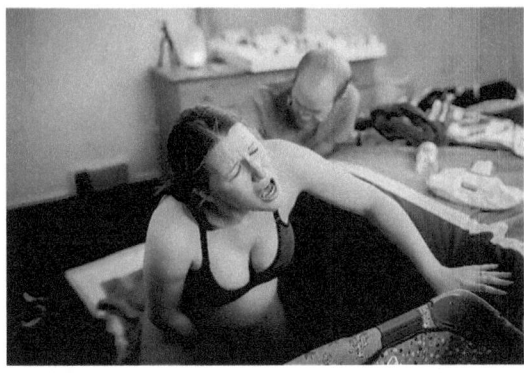

photo credit: Utah Birth Stories Photo + Film

This part gets super gross. Every contraction I had a bowel movement, very soft stool a bit like diarrhea. My husband grabbed a package of wipes and I would use them after every contraction because it was just too gross to leave it on my bottom. I said something about it being so gross and my husband and birth photographer both laughed, but I asked them not to laugh. I was working hard, and I didn't want to feel like I was being made fun of! To their credit, they both said some really supportive things and didn't laugh at me again.

I shifted from all fours to an upright lunge and back again, rocking back and forth, thrusting out my pelvis, willing that baby to come down, come out, and let it all be over. My hands were inside myself, wishing I could pull myself open all the way and let the baby out. I'm bellowing, making sounds I've never made before except in birth, in my mind I sound like a whale or a hippo, a large animal making intense sounds with each wave of contractions.

His head comes down, and I pant for a moment before pushing. I know I'm pushing too hard, I can feel it, but I can't wait any more. No patience left in me for another contraction. I don't want to wait, I want my baby here. I'm upright, feeling his head, feeling myself stretch, and it's only one or two pushes before his head is out, and then his body comes next and I catch him, my husband's hand on my hand helping our baby into this world.

My husband brings him down behind me, and I immediately ask for my baby. I want him now! The relief is immense. I'm so tired, so exhausted, so done. I hold my baby, who is fat and adorable and screaming.

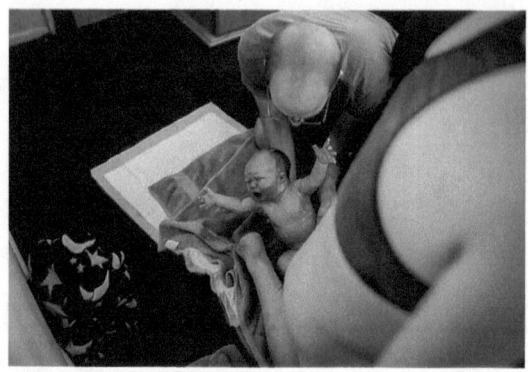

photo credit: Utah Birth Stories Photo + Film

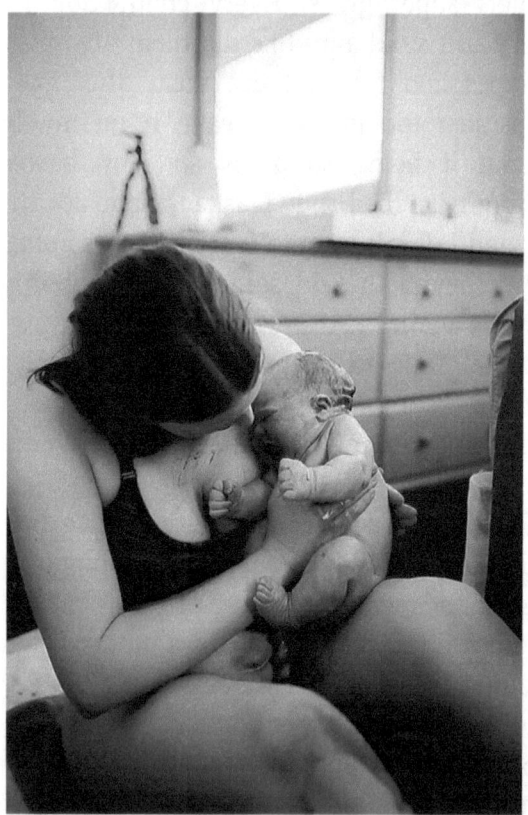

photo credit: Utah Birth Stories Photo + Film

I soak up those early moments, knowing that too soon they'll be gone, the vernix will be rubbed into his skin, his cord will be cut, and we will be two instead of one. Right now we are one, and I want to be warm.

We make our way to the bed and nurse for the first time. He's a champion breastfeeder. I admire his perfect fingers and toes, the warmth of his body on mine, his bright, alert eyes. He's here, our little boy.

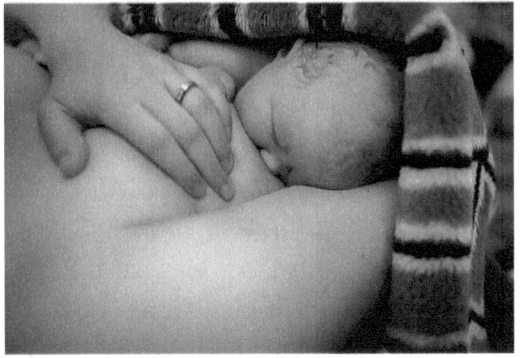

photo credit: Utah Birth Stories Photo + Film

After some time, I decide to get out of bed and attempt to birth the placenta. It hasn't come yet, but my bleeding is fine. I've taken some Angelica tincture to encourage it to come out, but nothing. Getting some strong afterbirth contractions with baby's nursing, too! WM husband does the honors, of cutting the cord and we clamp it with a regular plastic clamp, since we had one leftover after my previous birth. Handing off the baby to my husband, I climb out of bed and squat over a bowl while they weigh the baby.

10 lbs 3 oz, they announce. No wonder it was so hard! So much harder than my previous birth, which was 3 hours start to finish and the baby 2 lbs smaller than this one! Oh my goodness, this baby was a giant! I still feel such a sense of pride and gratitude when I realize I did that. With God, I grew and birthed a perfect 10 lb baby boy, our little Andrew. Ultimately, it took 41 weeks and 8 hours of labor to bring him here. He's calm and healthy and all around delightful, and I'm so grateful to have him here!

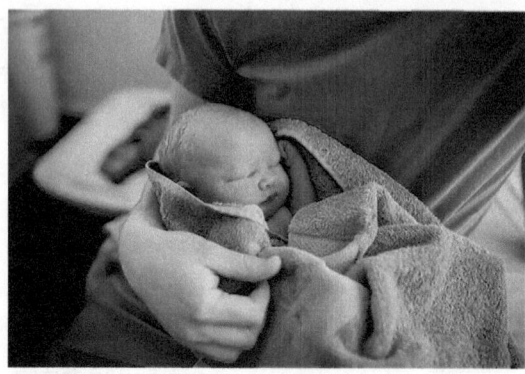

photo credit: Utah Birth Stories Photo + Film

To avoid sugar-coating it, this labor was hard. Possibly my hardest labor ever, and I've given birth five times now. I've taken self-hypnosis, I've done fear-clearings and energy healing, I've prayed and visualized my ideal birth, and this birth still brought me to my knees. Who knows why some births are orgasmic and others are painful enough to rock your soul? I won't pretend to be an expert. I think sometimes it's luck and sometimes it's something like fate. Either way, I believe that we have the pregnancies and labors and births that are meant to teach us and grow us the most. And if that's the case, then I trust that this labor was that for me. It taught me something I'm still trying to figure out. Some of it faith, some of it trust, some of it…something more about myself. My strength, my husband's strength, God's power and that He'll be there. Even if He doesn't change the outcome, He's there, and He knows our pain perfectly.

My husband and I have always talked about having eight kids. Honestly, it took an entire month after this baby before I admitted that I didn't feel done having children. This experience rocked me, but it didn't break me. It felt like I was giving birth for the first time again, and was the closest I've ever come to feeling traumatized by birth, but I emerged knowing I am capable of so much more than I give myself credit for.

My postpartum healing has gone really well. I made lots of preparation beforehand to ensure that I would have several weeks of complete support before I was left alone with all my kids and a house to maintain. That ended up being a huge blessing because I did tear with this one. You can read about my experience with healing my first-degree tear naturally in the coming chapters. I can say now, however, that everything healed wonderfully ,and at the time of this writing ,I'm six weeks postpartum and feeling pretty grand about everything down there.

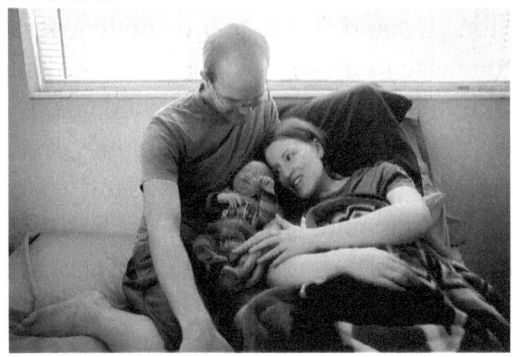

photo credit: Utah Birth Stories Photo + Film

Those are my stories. From hospital to my fifth freebirth, it's been quite a journey. I hope to have a few more babies, and a few more stories to tell. I hope they can be freebirths as well, I wouldn't have it any other way. (Since the original publication of this book, I've had my sixth baby and fourth freebirth. You can read about it in another collection of stories titled *Apricity: Bright Birth Stories for Winter's Dark*, available on Amazon.)

There's so much power in claiming birth. It's my greatest hope with the stories that follow that you will be able to claim your births for yourself and help others do the same.

So, why did I choose freebirth? Because freebirth made all the difference. It didn't make it less painful. It didn't really make it easier. What differences did I notice?

Having so much silence was freeing. Not literal silence, but the absence of anything that could interrupt my flow, my feeling of authority.

My husband was there, and that was it. He deferred to me completely. There was no perceived authority to distract or confuse his ability to respond fully to my needs.

I didn't have any expectations to meet, no imposed deadlines, limitations, or fears from anyone outside myself. No one was there to suggest things contrary to my intuition. Essentially, the biggest difference iwa the silencing of all outside voices, allowing the inner voice and feeling to be heard loud and clear.

Why not have a midwife? In freebirth, there is no other recognized authority besides the birthing woman. In preparing for my freebirths I became the authority in my labors. I could move into any position, eat or drink, use the bathroom and even have sex during labor without inhibition. I could listen to my body completely, without input from anyone else to make me doubt what my intuition told me. I also wasn't entertaining anyone, so I could make any sound, do anything, say anything I needed. I felt completely free.

When I felt fear, I could work with myself to push through. I relied on myself and the quiet strength of my husband, who is a true rock and support for me during my labors. There were times I felt fear or wondered what to do, but ultimately I could sense whether I needed further assistance (I didn't) or not. Experiencing that level of trust as a couple creates an incredible bond.

Some women choose freebirth for lack of options. I'm fortunate to live somewhere that all types of midwives are legal, giving me a full range of options. I still choose freebirth and will always choose freebirth, so long as my intuition tells me all is well with my body and my baby.

Lack of options doesn't always mean midwives aren't available, but perhaps they're financially out of reach. Insurance most often doesn't cover home birth options even when they exist, and though midwives are valuable and worth paying, it's not always within reach. Surprise pregnancies, financial hardship, and many other situations make saving up for midwifery care little more than a dream for some couples. I don't think it's responsible for this to be the only reason for a woman to choose freebirth. There must also be an emotional and mental component of readiness.

Freebirth isn't just a way to save a buck. It's a perk, certainly. My most freebirth expensive birth (the first one, where I bought all of my equipment including a sling scale, handheld Doppler, blood pressure cuff, etc. and hired a Doula, all well worth the cost) was roughly $650. My least expensive freebirth was this most recent one, with costs for supplies being less than $100, although I did see a chiropractor and massage therapist in addition.

Suffice it to say, freebirths can cost you very little, but that shouldn't be your main motivation for having one. Freebirth isn't for everyone, just as cesarean sections aren't for everyone. If you feel led to freebirth, then by all means, embark on the path; but listen closely to your intuition and follow it when it tells you that you need to seek assistance.

I will say, too, that there's no going back. Once you know what it's like to have true autonomy in birth, even watching assisted home birth with midwives becomes hard. You see just how much they interfere, how much their "noise" interrupts mother's intuition and bonding with her baby. Having an assisted birth no longer makes sense when you truly can do it yourself in most instances. Unless your intuition speaks otherwise, you may find that you never return to assisted childbirth.

Space and Support

WE MOVED DURING MY 5th pregnancy. I knew it would be a possibility, but we weren't certain we could sell our home and find a new home in the short time span we had available. My husband's new job had a terrible commute, and while we could have made it work longer, everything started to fall together with a home that fell into our laps and eager buyers that made selling our home much easier than we expected. So, at 35 weeks pregnant, we moved.

Not knowing where your birth space will be, and being unable to prepare or nest is stressful, to say the least. The month during and after our move I felt completely ungrounded. I tried self-hypnosis, eating well, drinking nourishing tea, speaking affirmations, talking out my feelings, but I never gained the sense of stability I longed for.

At the time of this writing I'm 40 weeks pregnant, and my emotions are still scattered. I'm trying to gather them in, to move past survival mode and get into a solid place I feel safe to give birth from. I realize that one thing keeping me from grounding is trying to decide where I want to give birth.

At home is the obvious choice. I have no desire to birth anywhere else, although if I am honest my dream would be for me to go into complete seclusion in a cozy space somewhere, away from the needs of my four young children, the stress of my husband, and everything that doesn't flow or function around this old (new) house.

So I wander from room to room, sometimes with the intent to put a few things in order or empty a moving box, and I try to visualize birthing there. Everything is still cluttered and not in its right place, so I find this visualization difficult, like riding a bike for the first time, or a playing an instrument again after many years. Nothing feels like "mine" yet. The entire house is in transition, from theirs to ours. I feel like a visitor, I don't feel comfortable, and I can't "see" where to give birth.

The master bedroom is close. It's small, but cozy, and feeling more ours the more time we spend in it. I put up the pack n' play. It's our sleeper of choice for when baby isn't co-sleeping in bed with me all the time, although it mostly gets used like a bedside stand and for holding baby stuff. I found a place for my nursing rocker, which, again, won't get used much until after the first few weeks. Maybe I'll birth in the bedroom. It's where my fourth baby was born, back at our previous home. It's where we make love, and that makes it easy to relax and let go.

I drop the items where they go (for now) and move on. I pass the front sitting room and kitchen. They feel too open, too exposed in this house. I may labor in one or the other, but they don't have the right feel for birth. I'm not planning a water birth, since I don't prefer them, so I pass the upstairs bathroom as well. I gravitate downstairs.

Navigating the steep and narrow staircase makes my heart pound this late in pregnancy. I worry about slipping and falling, but take it slow and make myself let go of those fears. The laundry room is an obvious no, although the large space would be the perfect place for a birthing tub if I cared for a water birth. There's a small den-like room, with a fireplace and, for now, random furniture cluttered against the walls. It has a private feel, but so sparse. I imagine ways I could make it feel cozier, more like a birthing space, and continue through to the next room.

It's a large living room, which we'll be using as a playroom. Lots of toys scattered on the floor right now, and there's an attached kitchen. The previous owners rented the basement. I like it, but it's too open, and like the den, too sparse. I can't see myself here. There's a bathroom with a closet-like shower between the den and the playroom. I take a deep breath and picture pushing my baby out there in various positions, maybe using the shower sometime in early labor. I might like it.

I head back upstairs. Most of this takes place at night, when my children are asleep. Sometimes, when they're awake and playing well together, I close my eyes and let my mind wander the halls of our new home, letting my mind work through different labor scenarios, even ones that seem ludicrous or strange. I'm often interrupted, but even so I sense myself getting closer to knowing what I want my labor space to be.

Take time to picture it. Especially if you're in a transient situation, when it might seem hard or even impossible to know exactly where you give birth, create words and feelings you want your space to have. How does it feel? My main word is comfortable, also safe and cozy. What kind of lighting would you like? Is a water birth important to you?

In visualizing your birth space, it's important to imagine your wildest dream birth space, as well as the more practical space. How can you invite the feeling of your dream birth space into the space you have to work with? Will having a certain person there help? Will having no one there help? Do you need some blankets, pillows, a salt lamp or twinkle lights? Maybe a streamer filled with written, drawn, or printed birthing affirmations would make it feel right. Or you could create a portable "altar", a tray filled with crystals and gems, pictures, candles, anything you feel drawn to use to support you in your labor. You can place these items where you know you'll give birth, if you know, or you can make it possible to carry them with you even if you change rooms.

Not everyone feels safe or comfortable having a freebirth at home, and the reasons for this vary. Maybe you live with someone who isn't supportive of home birth, much less freebirth. Maybe you don't have a permanent home. Maybe you're between homes. Maybe you just don't feel inclined to birth in the space you live in. Whatever the situation, you have every right to feel comfortable and safe. What will it take to get you there?

One benefit of freebirth is being able to give birth anywhere. I've heard of women giving birth in yurts in the mountains, trailers, small homes, the suburbs, outside in backyards or special places in the woods, in the ocean, in the desert, in hotels or airbnbs, even in the home of a friend or supportive family member. One of my friends planning a freebirth gave birth (to her surprise) in the bathroom of a formal dining restaurant! You can read her story in this book.

Where are you drawn to give birth? If it's not where you live, is there a place you can rent nearby? Do you have a friend who would let you birth in their space? I've seen women ask on social media platforms and find spaces to birth in provided by strangers, people who open their homes to those who want a place to give birth without judgement or fear.

At the end of the day, where you give birth isn't of great importance. You might prepare the most incredible, sacred-feeling birth space, only to push your baby out on the toilet. You might wander from state to state your entire pregnancy and end up in a cozy home of your own at the end. There's no right way, and there's no right space. Find what fits you and this birth. If, like me, you find yourself at the end of your pregnancy and still feeling ungrounded, find things that can anchor you to your ideal feeling for your birth, even if you can't find a space to be anchored to until the contractions begin.

An important part of your birthing space, more important than how it looks or where it is, is who you choose to have present. The next section will cover this vital component of freebirth.

Determining Your Birth Support

There is no wrong way to give birth. Some women want a full circle around them. Others want to be left completely alone. Many people will say that if a woman has someone at her birth other than herself or her husband, it "doesn't count" as freebirth.

Unassisted doesn't mean unsupported.

Every woman deserves as much support as she desires in her birth, freebirth or otherwise. In an ideal world, women would have access to every kind of support without being judged or harmed for her preferences. Unfortunately, we don't live in an ideal world. We live in an imperfect world. A world where you have to create your own circle of support, especially when you freebirth.

For my own freebirths, I've chosen to have a friend, Doula, or birth photographer at each one. They serve as an extra set of hands to fetch things or watch my children, and they are knowledgeable about and comfortable with birth. They are not a pseudo-midwife. They are not a cheap doctor. They are support. An extra set of hands. It's irresponsible to expect a birth professional who is not medically trained to support you medically, and if you're hiring or asking a Doula to be at your birth so that someone with more knowledge than you is there, that is not the right motivation for having her there. It will put both you and the Doula in a very uncomfortable position should an emergency occur and you expect more of her than she can offer.

So what can a Doula do? As a Doula that attends unassisted births myself, I can tell you that a Doula will most likely provide the following:

- Comfort measures such as rebozo, massage, counter pressure, aromatherapy, etc.
- Contributing knowledge about pregnancy, birth, and postpartum and where to find answers (they will not give not medical advice)
- Childcare and pre-birth education for your kids (sibling Doula)
- Book recommendations, possibly a whole lending library
- Emotional support for you and your partner

Doulas won't usually do vaginal exams, use dopplers, catch babies, cut cords, or give medical advice. If you want someone to do those things, don't have a freebirth.

If you want a Doula to do something but aren't sure she will, just ask.

Also, don't be surprised if it's difficult to find a Doula in your area who isn't afraid of the potential liability in attending an unassisted birth. The risk of said liability is tiny, but a critical deal-breaker for some Doulas, depending on their certifying agency. Most likely they are not a good fit for you anyway, if this is the case.

Despite how hard it might be to find a Doula to support your freebirth should you want one, do not, under any circumstance, hide your plans to freebirth. Your relationship with your Doula relies on trust. It's better to make your plans clear from the start and ask for referrals if the Doula you talk to isn't inclined to support you. Otherwise, you might find that they drop you as a client, refuse to attend your birth, or even call 911 without your permission, and who would blame them? It's your responsibility to make sure everyone at your birth supports you completely.

A Doula is not a midwife. Your friend is not a midwife. Your husband is not a midwife.

When you freebirth, you become your own midwife. You may have people there to help, but you must put it in your mind that the responsibility to understand pregnancy, birth, and when to transfer to the hospital is all yours. You should determine who catches your baby either yourself, your husband, or someone else. You should be prepared to make the judgement call to phone 911 should it become necessary. You should be the authority at your own birth. If anyone else is calling the shots, that defeats the purpose of freebirth.

The following are some red flags that may indicate that someone you've invited to attend your birth isn't truly supportive:

- Do they often ask whether you plan to receive prenatal testing, appointments, or ultrasounds, even after you've told them no?
- Do they try to pressure or guilt you into anything you are not comfortable with?
- Do they make statements that cause you to feel bad or ashamed about your choices?
- Do you leave conversations with them doubting your choices and your ability to give birth?
- Do they seem to fear birth more than they respect your choices?

You may choose to see a medical provider, either midwife or doctor, during your pregnancy. You may choose to receive some testing. You may even choose to hire a non-medical provider to be at your birth to help out in some form or another. All of these situations still qualify you for freebirth. It's not about who is at your birth or whether you receive a medicalized model of prenatal care. It's about you, and how free you are to make the choices that need to be made. It's about following your intuition without pressure from the emotions or "knowledge" of others clouding your way. It's about autonomous birth.

So, be honest with yourself: are you hiring (or inviting) this person, whether care provider or family or friend, to be at your birth because you do not trust yourself to know when assistance is needed? Are they there to replace your intuition? This may be one sign that you're not prepared for freebirth.

Giving Birth Alone

I can't speak to this from personal experience. There was a brief time of perhaps ten minutes in my fourth birth (second freebirth) when my husband felt the energy in the room shift and felt strongly he should leave my side and give me the opportunity to labor alone. I felt every minute of those contractions acutely, and wished he would come back. I'm not sure what purpose it served, but I sense that I progressed rather fast in those minutes that he was gone. In my third freebirth, I went to the bathroom alone and labored down for a while, also furthering progress without anyone else present. Sometimes being alone is what your body needs.

The important thing is that you choose what feels best to you. I have always found it helpful to have an extra set of hands to catch my babies. I'm often too lost in labor land to bring myself to guide them into the world, and it has been a special, sweet bonding experience to have my husband do it. With my third freebirth, my husband and I caught our baby together.

That said, it is possible to safely birth your babies without anyone else in the room. Some women make a soft nest for their babies to land in. Other women birth in the water where it's easier to maneuver yourself and catch your baby.

Considerations for support would depend on whether you feel you need someone to watch older children, or desire someone to be there to hand you things that you can't get to, or provide comfort measures for labor (like counterpressure, rebozo sifting, massage, etc.). My placentas have been a bit sticky after my freebirths, requiring me to move around to get them out, and it was nice to have someone there to hold the baby and keep them warm while I worked on my placenta.

If you ask my husband, he'll tell you that it's nice to have a third set of hands to help with these things.

Speaking of spouses…are you wondering how to convince yours that freebirth is safe? Then the next chapter is for you!

Getting Your Spouse or Partner On-board

GETTING YOUR BIRTH PARTNER on board is one of the most-asked questions in freebirth circles. I remember when I first brought the idea to my husband before the birth of our third baby. I had been interviewing midwives but didn't feel great about any of them. We'd had a home birth before, but with a midwife. I knew he was already comfortable with home birth, which was a big help, but he was TERRIFIED of the idea of an unassisted birth. When I first told him I was considering it, my super-supportive baby-catching husband stared at me with wide eyes and said, "But what if you DIED?"

"What if I died? How likely is that to happen?" Was my reply. He didn't know, and together we researched until we found a statistic for maternal mortality in birth in the United States. I think the biggest shock for him was seeing that all the countries higher than us were third-world countries without access to medical care. And that a lot of European countries were WAY ahead of us with low maternal mortality rates, and they tend to value midwifery care models for the majority of women.

He didn't agree right then. He was, frankly, overwhelmed, so I let it go. I let the seed get planted, and then I watered it occasionally. I read everything I could get my hands on, every freebirth story, researched every emergency and how to deal with it. We would be sitting together doing our separate thing after the older two kids were in bed and I would just show him a quick statistic, or ask him how he would react if the baby were breech. I talked to him as if we were having an unassisted birth, I stopped looking for midwives.

Essentially, I acted as if he had already said yes and gave him time and space to figure his own emotions out.

One night, I was about halfway through my pregnancy, I asked him what he thought about it and he said that he trusted me. He was still afraid, but he trusted me to be prepared with the knowledge and tools needed. He also asked me to help educate him, which was incredibly humble of him. He asked me to tell him exactly what he would need to do to help me. And he wanted a Doula, another person there just to be an additional set of hands in case he was busy helping me and we needed something fetched or someone to be with the kids.

There are resources throughout this book, websites, podcasts, and books that you can use to persuade your partner to come with you on this freebirth journey.

When you've already decided you want a freebirth, it can be hurtful when he initially says no, especially if he acts like you're crazy or starts spouting his fears. Take a deep breath and ask him why he feels that way. You might be surprised by the answer. Just listen, don't respond. Communication 101: Too many people hear what the other has to say and then jump down their throat with a response without validating the other person's opinion. Instead, listen carefully and repeat back what they say as calmly as you can manage. For example:

You: I want to birth this baby at home without a midwife. No doctor, no hospital.

Him: No way. That's crazy. We're not doing that.

You: Why do you feel that way? What is your biggest fear?

Hopefully, he responds with at least one reason. "The baby could die. You could die. What if you bleed everywhere? What if you tear?" Those are a few of the most common ones. He might not give you much insight and just repeat his refusal. If that happens, you could use this line:

Do you have any evidence that supports the hospital being the safest place for me to give birth?

Most likely he doesn't. He might bring up a relative he knows that almost died or whose baby had complications. The best thing to do in this situation is to ask, "Do you know how likely it is that X complication will occur?" Again, he probably doesn't. Don't make him feel ignorant, just gently help him come to a realization of his own ignorance. You could ask him if he would watch a documentary with you, or if he'd be open to seeing statistics about that specific complication.

Sometimes it's better to end the conversation there, as frustrating as it is for you, and to address it another time. Even then, you might respond to one fear he has and another one will come up. Be patient as you work with him. This might mean that you have to compromise for a little while, like attending prenatal visits with a care provider you don't intend to birth with. Or, especially if your partner isn't very involved with the details of your pregnancy, you could start your own prenatal care and begin to act as if your plan to birth unassisted is going to come to fruition.

I have to add that I fully recognize that not all relationships are based on the mutual respect and understanding needed to work through fears and objections in this way. Sometimes partners are toxic, abusive, or manipulative, and even bringing up the subject could be dangerous to you physically or emotionally. If this is the case for you, please evaluate why you are in this relationship and whether it is even safe for you to stay. You might need to consider getting help to leave and finding another place to birth your baby.

"If the marriage is strong before the birth, it is likely that a newfound tenderness occurs after the birth. Lovers observe each other in new ways and new revelations are made. Husbands and wives usually experience a greater bonding. The yearning to become visible in your beloved's eyes will be felt the moment a new addition arrives in your family. It's magical, mystical, and divine. The visibility that is most meaningful is the shared event that takes place inside the family bubble, an historical moment best experienced in private. It is an ordinary, yet extraordinary life event between two lovers."

For a more comprehensive presentation of this topic, please refer to the book "Unassisted home birth: An Act of Love."

That isn't to say that all partners who say "no" to freebirth are abusive. It is far more likely that he is afraid. He's afraid of the "what if", the terrifying unknown. If you've had a previous birth inside the medical model that he witnessed, he may have experienced second-hand trauma that he never dealt with. He may be afraid that the same thing will happen again, or that it could be worse.

On the other hand, if nothing went "wrong" in his eyes during a hospital or midwife-led experience in the past, he may think it's illogical for you to want a different experience. This was the camp my husband fell into. We'd had a wonderful experience with a midwife at home before, so why would I want anything different? At the time all I could tell him was that it felt right and that none of the midwives I interviewed seem to have my interests truly at heart. For so many men, living in the logical side of their brains, feeling something is right isn't an entirely valid reason to make a critical life decision.

In the end, if your partner doesn't commit to your vision of a birth without assistance, you have three choices:

Compromise

It's not ideal. Some would argue it's completely dis-empowering to give up your autonomy and ignore your intuition. But there are situations where it may be the best option. I can't tell you what those situations are. That is for you alone to decide, and the situations vary so widely it wouldn't be fair to assign certain situations to the category of compromise. Just know that it is a valid path to take and that you can still have a wonderful, even autonomous birth experience.

Try to find out where your partner's comfort level is, and try to stretch it and help him grow. Maybe he just doesn't want to be the only one there. Your compromise could be to have a Doula, midwife, or traditional birth attendant on call as someone with more knowledge about birth.

Maybe home birth midwives aren't widely available in your area or even legal, or he'd rather you not birth at home. Your compromise could be to birth at a birth center, preferably free-standing, but if that's not available then a more naturally-minded hospital would be your next step.

If he is very fear-driven or being heavily influenced by the fears of friends, coworkers, or family, he may insist that you give birth at the hospital, and if there are no hospitals known for being supportive of natural options, you may find yourself in a rather tight spot, trying to find an obstetrician that supports autonomous birth but is still covered by insurance because hospital birth is expensive. That alone might be a point that persuades your loved one to support your birth at home if you mention that the only care provider or hospital you'll give birth with is out-of-network.

If there's one thing that speaks well to men in the absence of all other reasoning, it's money. Freebirth is free. You can give birth with just yourself and a towel, no other equipment needed. There are things that make it a little nicer, cleaner, more convenient, but nothing you truly need beyond yourself. You actually don't even need your partner, but you may want him there. Remind him of this, of your love for him and for the child you've created together, then give it time. A compromise early in your pregnancy might soften his heart enough that he agrees later on.

It's up to you how far you're willing to take the compromise, but you'll get further convincing him of your desires the more you pour on love and respect in every conversation with him about where to give birth and with whom.

My Body, My Birth

Or, in other words, "No uterus, no opinion." This baby is growing inside YOUR body. What happens during pregnancy and birth has physical and emotional ramifications for you that can last throughout the rest of your life. Is that something you're willing to compromise in the face of someone else's fear?

This isn't just about you, it's about your baby and your family. Standing your ground in where and how you give birth can lead to new levels of respect and love in your marriage once you're on the other side of the experience. Emilee Saldaya of the Freebirth Society Podcast is one of the biggest advocates of making sure your partner understands and respects that birth is your domain, and therefore your decision. She says, "Never let your partner's fear of birth ruin your right to birth freely."

Remember that your husband can't stop labor once it has started. He has no power in the face of Mother Nature. The most he can do is call 911, and even then you will give birth, and you can give birth in the way you see fit or you can give in to his fear, the emergency personnels' fears, and do whatever they say regardless of your own confidence and intuition. The choice is ultimately yours.

I encourage using the utmost respect as you express this to your partner. It can be very inflammatory in a relationship and your partner could feel disrespected, disregarded, shutout, and angry.

Using your autonomy in this way will bring up all sorts of emotion, so be prepared. Your partner might seem to agree, or at least not fight you on it, and then lose his cool when it comes time for you to give birth. He might also get angry and it could be a source of stress and contention the rest of your pregnancy, creating an toxic environment for labor. He is your partner; you wouldn't be with him unless you loved him, and he's the other parent for your baby, so consider that he feels concern for the baby, concern for you, and that he's doing the best he can to protect both of you with his current knowledge and understanding.

Having this attitude might seem inflammatory, but consider the reality of birth. It's absolutely your domain, your birthright. No one can give birth for you, though in the hospital they often try. Birth is YOURS, and if you step fully into that it will cause shockwaves going forward and backward in your genealogical line, healing mistreatment women have undergone at the hands of men (and other women) essentially since the beginning of time. This is you in all your divine, feminine strength.

If you do tell him it's your body, your decision and go on to attempt freebirth, there are a few things that could happen:

1. He could call 911 while you're in labor without your consent, leading strangers to barge in and insist you go to the hospital while you're in the throes of labor
2. He could stand around paralyzed, spouting fear and being generally unhelpful
3. He could jump into action and actually end up participating exactly the way you hoped.

What it really comes down to is, are you willing to risk that he might call 911 and end up disrupting your entire birth experience? If not, consider this as a truly last resort.

UNINVITE HIM

Just what it sounds like. Whether you tell him to his face or not, you have the power to uninvite him from your birth. It IS your body, and it IS ultimately your decision. Make plans to birth at a friend's house, hotel room, or just not tell him when you're in labor and try to birth quietly in a distant part of the house if he's home. This option relies on the belief that "it's easier to ask forgiveness than permission." It also depends on finding a space to birth, or him either being a heavy sleeper, frequent traveler, or at work when you go into labor, so it's definitely not foolproof.

I caution the use of this option on two counts: first, your relationship might never recover once he finds out. And second, it's REALLY nice to have a second pair of hands helping when you're in labor! Yes, women can and do give birth completely by themselves, sometimes even outside in the wild. Personally, however, I appreciate having my husband give me hip squeezes, gather birth or postpartum supplies, hold the baby while I birth the placenta, and bring water or food as needed.

You could invite a supportive female attendant, friend, or family member to be with you during this time instead of your partner, but you should make it clear whether your partner is allowed in the room.

We love our men, but they don't always listen to us as well as… well, other men. Which is why I interviewed my husband for this next part. A little conversation from my guy to yours.

"Partner Talk" with Tyler Moore

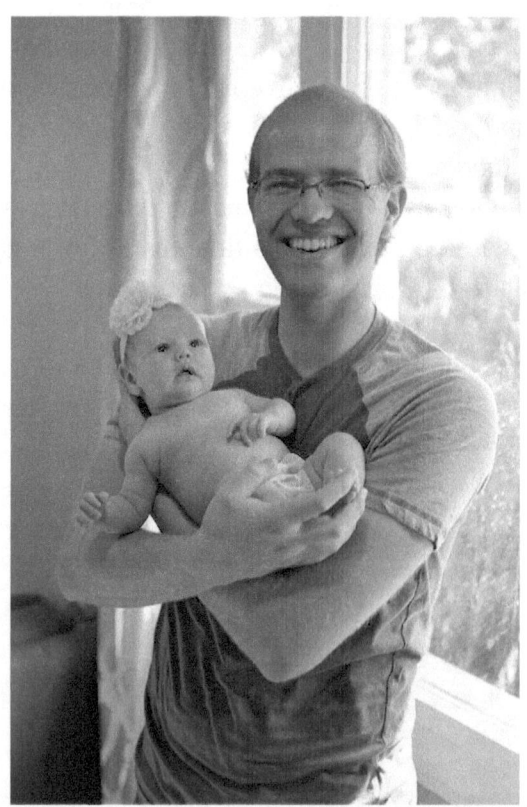

Tyler and Kaylee, our fourth baby, after our second freebirth.

Q: What were your first feelings when your wife told you she wanted to birth unassisted? How did you work through those emotions?

A: Since that first freebirth was with our third child, it really wasn't as scary anymore. Having already done two births, one at the hospital and one at home, there was a lot I already knew. I had already been through the process. The idea of doing it unassisted wasn't nearly as frightening as it could have been. The biggest preparation that I knew needed to happen was to have a plan in place for "what if" things go wrong, and how to know things were going wrong. As soon as we had that in place, it was easy. Also, seeing my wife and her cognizance giving birth, her awareness of her body and her ability to communicate during labor really also gave me a lot more confidence and assuaged a lot of my fears.

Q: What would you say are the most common fears or objections for men as they're confronted with their partner's radical birth choices?

A: Not knowing what's going to happen. Every birth you don't know. I mean, from the time the pregnancy starts, you don't know what the baby is going to do in the actual birth itself. Is the baby going to be head-down, facing the right direction? Is the baby going to refuse to turn and you're suddenly confronted with a breech birth? Or what happens if in the week leading up to the baby being born your wife says, "I don't feel baby moving as much?" What if something serious does go wrong and we can't make it to the hospital in time? That kind of stuff.

Is the place we're giving birth sanitary? For our first unassisted we were living in my grandmother's basement, which was kind of dingy. We also didn't have a door separating our space from hers, just knowing someone outside of the birth experience could be listening or walk in at any time, having that little bit of extra tension, it was a potential source of complication for me.

Q: What advice do you have for the father who is fearful for the well-being of his wife/partner and child during birth?

If it's the first birth, and she wants to go unassisted. Oh man! You have got to be willing to trust HER instinct or intuition or whatever you call it. If she says it's right for her, you better trust it and you better watch some unassisted birth videos so you know what's going on and what's expected of you. 'Cause if it's your first it's going to be 100% new and that will prevent you from being able to be there.

You have to know whether or not you CAN assist her. Because if you're watching these videos and you're puking or gagging or going pale at the sight of birth, then she's got to find someone else. Because if you can't help, you got to make sure she's got at least some support that she can rely on. We say it's "unassisted," but mom can't be superhuman. There will come a point in the birth - almost guaranteed - where she will say she's done and want to quit and that's when she needs to hear some words of encouragement and just needs a little bit of extra help.

Now, if it's not your first, hopefully you stuck around through the other births and you know what to expect. Then you need to prepare yourself to know the signs of problems, so that you can wisely assist.

Also, check the statistics. If you're into numbers. If you're more of a feelings person, take time to feel it out.

To men being domineering and flat-out refusing to "allow" their wives to freebirth, I say why? Why should you, a man, dictate what happens within the partnership of birth? It took two to make the baby, and it's going to take both to get the baby out. Don't let your pride destroy your wife, her dreams and her intuition.

Q: What do you/ did you tell others about your plans for giving birth at home without assistance? Did you ever meet resistance, fear, or skepticism? How did you handle that?

A: I didn't ever tell people until after we'd done it the first time. People would ask or show fear, kinda like "wait, isn't that dangerous?" "I've heard of that, but I would never do it myself." I would just assure them that I was well-educated, I knew what the signs were, I'd studied and was confident that I could recognize when there was a problem. I knew what to do if things did go wrong. We were ready, and we were okay calling 911 if things did turn south. Most people when they hear that will say, "Wow, that's brave, I would never do that." or "That's crazy! Put me in a hospital and give me an epidural and surround me with nurses." And, okay, cool. I once told a chiropractor who had done unassisted births with his wife. He said, "If I did not have my degree as a doctor of chiropractics I would not even consider it. Because I have medical training similar to a doctor, that's what gave me the confidence." That was a fun conversation!

I never really met resistance or criticism. Most people that I talk to understand that your birth is your birth, whatever you and your wife decide, it's your thing. I never had anyone try to talk me out of it. I think part of it is the progressive age that we're in; people don't interfere anymore. But I also tend to only tell people that already know that I'm a little bit different than normal. I play it safe. I don't just barge in and announce that I did an unassisted birth. If they're already iffy about a home birth, I don't mention that it was unassisted.

Q: Have any issues occurred during your births at home that gave you pause, made you afraid, or required you to do something unexpected?

A: Yes. During our third baby's birth, when her head first came out the cord ran at least across her neck. For half a second I thought "Oh crap, we're going to have to go to the ER." Of course, no. I knew I needed to check the tension in the cord. As soon as I knew it was really loose, I knew to let it be. Baby was getting plenty of blood. Sure enough, baby came out super easy. As she came out I moved the cord so it slid down her body and wouldn't tighten or get pulled. That baby also had an umbilical hernia and I didn't understand how that worked until a few days later, when I learned it's not a really big deal.

Q: What advice can you give women who are discouraged by their partner's/husband's lack of support in their desire for a freebirth?

A: This is the hardest question. I would ask, what form does the lack of support from your husband take? Is it domineering, or it an insecurity or fear? Is it rooted in a misunderstanding? Where is the lack of support coming from? See if you can help resolve those issues. See if you can present data, facts, videos, something to your husband, and see if it can answer their questions that they don't know they have.

If they refuse to look at the information you show them, you've got to start praying for them or asking them to trust you more. Even just to trust you enough to look at the stuff that you're showing them. See if it can help to change their hearts, their lack of support. That's step one: see where they're at, and help them to change it.

Step two is to talk to a friend who has done it. Intentionally sit in the room with your husband so he overhears it or is part of the conversation. Talk to other birth professionals and try to bring him along. Midwives who support freebirth. Doulas who support freebirth. Friends who have gone through it.

Understand your partner's fear. Help them understand their fear. Help them resolve their fear and bring in additional support. Tell them what you FEEL and what you THINK about freebirth. Use BOTH feelings and logic. If they're someone who goes with their gut, ask them what their gut says.

It's essential that the birthing mom and her partner agree on whatever course of action is being taken. Whether that means the husband agrees to be in the birthing space and helping, or be in the birthing space and not helping, or be out of the birthing space and letting the wife be alone or with another support. You have to both agree to whatever is going on and agree that no blame will exist between you should anything go wrong. It's a joint venture. Doesn't matter who the birthing partner is, you're partners for some reason, and so it's about maintaining a healthy relationship with that person. If you're going behind their back it can be devastating to a relationship.

Q: Do you think your experiences with freebirth changed your marriage/ relationship? How?

A: Yes. It taught me better to trust my wife. To let go sometimes of the preconceived notions, the ideas and things that I once thought were "the law", and be open to at least looking into and possibly trying out new things. So that you know for yourself if it's good. Just hearing sometimes isn't enough. Some things you have to experience for yourself. Doing that helped me to trust my wife. Because she was encouraging me to try new things, to reach out in a different direction, further than I'd reached before. I learned so many lessons from that.

For instance, it taught me to trust what my wife says for each of our independent births. The first two, she wanted me to touch her. The last one, my instinct said not to touch her, but I did anyway and she slapped my hand and told me not to touch her. I'm glad I listened to that because later she told me that it helped when I stopped touching her this time. There was no pattern to follow. The pattern was, "What does my wife need? What does she tell me she needs?"

Self-led Pregnancy

"Truly unhindered birth is birth without resistance; unhindered birth comes through learning to meet your body's needs throughout pregnancy, learning to listen to your baby…it comes through learning to identify when things are not right, and finding solutions. It comes through learning to identify your inner voice, and respecting that voice as your greatest authority."

- *Sarah M. Haydock, "Unhindered Childbirth: Wisdom for the Passage of Unassisted Birth"*

To Test or Not to Test

The first intervention is the pregnancy test, used by millions of women to "prove" or confirm a pregnancy. Many live or die to see that little pink line. It often brings reassurance, confidence, excitement, joy, and permission to begin care.

I have no qualms with pregnancy tests. I've used them with all five of my pregnancies, although I'm determined not to test if we have another baby. Why? There's no risks. It's not invasive. And yet, I wonder how we are limiting ourselves by needing something outside ourselves to say that we're pregnant, instead of sitting with not knowing and finding that confidence and joy for ourselves.

It's the first opportunity we get to practice intuition. It's our first encounter with not knowing, and instead, waiting for our wise bodies to reveal the truth in their own time. It becomes harder to build this intuition the more we rely on outside influences to give us arbitrary knowledge about the state of our pregnant bodies.

Of course, taking a pregnancy test (or three!) in no way disqualifies you from freebirth. The whole point of freebirth is that you choose the care that you want and need without feeling pressure from anyone else to confirm or perform. What feels most true and right to you? That is what you do.

Unassisted Prenatal Care

I once heard someone say, "Prenatal care is the care that happens between prenatal visits." The sentiment is powerful. Wherever and with whomever you give birth, unassisted or not, most of your care should be given by yourself through diet, exercise, spiritual practices, etc. Any outside assistance you seek is supplemental to the care you give yourself, though many women often rely on medical prenatal care providers far too much. As if seeing a doctor or midwife once a month for a few moments of conversation and testing will magically grant one a perfectly healthy pregnancy and an ideal birth, and the equal and opposite belief, that missing such appointments could result in utter devastation of your or your unborn baby's health.

I started questioning the need for prenatal appointments in my first pregnancy, a planned hospital birth with a rotating practice of midwives. Appointments were inconvenient and annoying, riddled with uncomfortable situations like testing that I would have preferred to refuse (but didn't, because I was too busy playing the 'good girl' to act on my intuition), and the impersonal, too-short conversations with a different midwife each time (I wanted to get to know them all, since I didn't know who I would be seeing during labor).

I started wishing I could skip them. Looking back, I recognize my discomfort for what it was: the result of my compromise with my husband to have him support my preference for a completely unmedicated birth, at the expense of my desire to have a home waterbirth. He was too uncomfortable with the idea of a home birth, and it seemed far too expensive for our financial situation. So, I stayed with the midwives and I went to appointments and I shrugged off my discomfort so I could have what I wanted: a supported natural birth.

I got that experience, but the price was too high, and my next pregnancy was different. I still believed in the ritual of prenatal visits, more habit than anything at this point. I had read so much about pregnancy and birth there was little need to go to these appointments except to keep my husband and my midwife happy, so I went. Longer and much more personal, I almost looked forward to these appointments, except that there was a growing, subconscious sense that I wasn't the authority. I responded to the midwife's perceived authority more than my own inner authority. That response reflected in my birth experience when I tore terribly, ignoring my own signals in favor of 'getting the baby out,' which was my perception of what the midwife and everyone else in the room wanted me to do.

I interviewed two midwives for my third pregnancy. We had moved, so I couldn't use the midwife from my second birth, a blessing in disguise. I hired one, had my first prenatal visit with her, and was confronted with so much fear-mongering that I began to question everything this midwife asked me to do. I cancelled my next appointment, determined to have a freebirth. I am fortunate to have a husband who chose to trust me more than he feared the unknowns of birth.

In order to counteract his fear and prove freebirth was safe, however, I mimicked the outline of the medicalized prenatal care I had received in the past. We bought a blood pressure cuff and learned how to use it, a Doppler and fetoscope, a tape measure to check fundal height, and so on. The only thing I didn't get was urine strips, because I didn't see much point in them to begin with. I faithfully tracked all measurements for me and our baby on a spreadsheet on the computer each month. My husband was my stand-in midwife, taking most of my measurements as a way of being involved. The birth was wonderful.

My fourth pregnancy I became even more relaxed. The Doppler came out a handful of times, and then we switched to the fetoscope (I was gradually coming to an awareness of the harms of Doppler waves on a growing unborn baby). I checked fundal height and my blood pressure every now and then, just to have a baseline should something happen later in the pregnancy, but far less than monthly. I rarely remembered prenatal vitamins, only taking them if my intuition indicated I needed to. I supplemented the medical model of prenatal care with my own model of intuitive care. The birth was fast and again, wonderful.

In my fifth pregnancy, you could hardly find a trace of medicalized prenatal care. Except for a single doppler check in the first trimester, and an ultrasound at 22 weeks (which I regret, to some degree), I have made my prenatal care more about intuition than ever before. Now and then I'll step on a scale, when it's convenient (since we don't own one), and when I'm in the mood I'll pull out the measuring tape and check my fundal height, but never for anything other than curiosity's sake.

Thoughts on Nutrition

I generally try to eat healthy, but avoid extremes in pregnancy diet. I eat what feels and sounds good, I don't limit any food group in particular, and if I start to feel unwell, I double check what I've eaten recently and increase foods that are high in nutrients I might be lacking.

Nutrition is definitely important during pregnancy, but I'll be the first to say that so is following your intuition. Find balance between getting enough nutrients and eating what sounds and feels good to you. Now is not the time to start a diet or dramatically change what you eat unless you feel inspired and uplifted by the change, rather than guilted into it.

In Laura Kaplan Shanley's Book "Unassisted Childbirth," she discusses how it's the beliefs about what we're eating that are more damaging than the actual nutritional content of our food, and how an intuitive woman will be able to let go of false beliefs and enjoy all kinds of food without judgement or shame towards herself or her body. Truly an ideal to strive for, and far more important than whether we eat strictly vegan or enough vegetables or abstain from all sugar.

Pregnancy is a time to indulge in the abundance the earth has given, and that includes both sweet and savory.

> "The fact is most people assign far too much power to food, and far too little power to their own minds."
>
> - Laura Kaplan Shanley

THOUGHTS ON EXERCISE

I didn't exercise much during any of my pregnancies, and this one least of all. Between my fourth and fifth pregnancies, I experienced a pelvic floor imbalance resulting in severe right-side hip pain that would flare up after exercise of any duration or intensity. Chiropractic, energy work, massage, heat and ice, essential oils, and muscle balancing exercises all did nothing. The only way I avoided pain was by avoiding extreme physical activity, which for me meant anything outside my typical daily movement. I practiced trust in my body, knowing that my inner wisdom is far more important to follow than the scientific claims about the amount of exercise one should do during pregnancy. I felt healthy, I felt balanced, I felt calm and knew that all would be well.

Aside from what I've mentioned already, my prenatal care included the occasional chiropractic visit, a couple massages, and some hypnosis and meditation to prepare for birth. My focus and investment has been on ensuring I'll have the support I need to heal properly after this birth, something I value immensely.

So, my two-bits on prenatal care is that it can be whatever you make it. I have a more relaxed approach. Some women prefer, for various reasons, to remain with a medical provider for prenatal care, rather than going completely unassisted throughout their pregnancy. Whatever you choose, let it be out of confidence, and follow your intuition.

My one warning about unassisted prenatal care is that there is such a thing as being TOO lax. Ignoring warning signs and avoiding the diagnoses the medical institution can give because of fears, prejudice, or past trauma can be dangerous. I'm not saying every little symptom should mean a trip to the emergency room, but judicious and intuitive use of modern medicine has its place. If you think you might want to seek care but don't want to go in for what ends up being nothing, ask yourself the ultimate question: what will you do if something turns out to be wrong?

Pretend in your mind that you choose to seek care. You go in, and what can they offer you? If you think you're miscarrying, they can give you a vaginal exam, a Doppler reading, and an ultrasound to confirm or deny the miscarriage. If you're far enough along (past 25 or so weeks), they might offer to attempt to stop labor if they think they will succeed or that your baby will survive. In this situation, you must weigh whether having the certainty of knowing if you are miscarrying will outweigh the possible trauma that could come from your treatment at the hospital, which will depend largely on the attitude and demeanor of the nurses and doctors you encounter.

Or, you could choose to let go of the illusion of control and sit with not knowing. It's uncomfortable, isn't it? Not knowing. But it's something you will run into throughout your pregnancy, and perhaps most especially at the end. At the time I'm writing this, I am roughly 38 weeks pregnant with my fifth baby. In past pregnancies, I've given birth as early as 40+1 and as late as 42+3, not that due dates hold much water in my book. I've been aching for this baby to be born since 34 weeks, which means that despite knowing I could have two months left, part of me wondered if it would happen sooner, if it could happen sooner. I've had to sit with that 'not knowing', and let it go.

As long as I choose autonomous birth, I will never know the exact day my babies will be born. I've been decent at guessing, but in the end, this person growing inside of me has a mind of his own and he will come when he is ready. Every tightening, every strange sensation, every shift of my body will have me wondering if today is the day. Each night I fall to sleep and each morning I wake up still pregnant brings a tiny wave of disappointment before I take a deep breath and gather my courage and stamina for another day of being pregnant and not knowing.

The tools of a medical care provider can offer nothing but a vague glimpse into a single moment of a pregnancy. The ultrasound you get today proves that in a window of time, your baby was well. The doppler-magnified heart rate proves that in a particular moment in time, your baby's heart was beating. A vaginal exam shows that right now, you are dilated x-amount, but in an hour or a day or a week, you could be giving birth and that vaginal exam would have no bearing on the outcome, unless you choose to take action from it, which far too many women do.

Women choose induction for being very dilated in the last weeks of pregnancy, as well as being 'too little' dilated. Impatience and fear control the decision in most cases.

Women choose to terminate pregnancies that ultrasounds and tests indicate aren't viable, or would result in deformity, death, or mental incapacity, despite the fact that both are shown to have high rates of false-positives.

Women choose cesarean for large babies, small babies, 'dying' placentas, twins, and many other situations that, given the evidence available, don't always indicate a need for automatic surgery.

And yet, women do. We buy into it all the time. We pay doctors and insurance companies large amounts of money to tell us, as often as possible, that everything is going right and we have nothing to fear. When we end up with a traumatic birth we thank them for being there, for saving us.

What if we bought into ourselves? What if we invested in our own care, our own intuition? What if we looked inside ourselves and found everything right and trusted that feeling, even in the face of miscarriage, deformity, death, and other less-desired outcomes? Can we accept that these things are part of our experience, part of our baby's experience, part of our mortal experience?

Doing so requires that we accept death as part of the life experience, which it is, irrevocably. None of us can avoid it, no matter how much organic food we eat, how much praying we do, how much medical care we do or don't get. All of us will die, and it is this truth, above all, that we have to be prepared to accept when we journey on the path to freebirth. We accept responsibility for our actions in the face of the knowledge that either way we choose, we choose to live the best life we know to be possible, whether it be long or short, whether our babies live or die, there is no right answer in pregnancy and birth. There is only acceptance.

What does your acceptance look like? What will help you most on your journey to the hoped-for outcome of a live, healthy baby and mother? It will be different for everyone. In this book and the others you read, you'll find resources for your customized prenatal care.

I've gotten most everything I've used for my own prenatal care at www.inhishands.com. I highly recommend this website. Though there are others, most have similar pricing and it's very affordable. That said, your prenatal care can cost as much or as little as you require or desire. There is nothing you NEED to buy, perhaps save food and drink, which are the most basic and necessary of care. But there are, maybe, things that you want, things that you feel drawn towards, and I encourage you to make a list and see how you can bring those things into your life no matter what your financial circumstances are.

THINKING IT'S TWINS?

Every pregnancy from my third on, I've had the thought, "Could this be twins?" It's a super common thought among multiparas (women who have given birth more than twice), and even more so among those choosing freebirth. Why would that be the case? Well, most freebirthers aren't going to the doctor to check heart rate via Doppler or have an early ultrasound (which is completely excessive and only used to "prove" the pregnancy and determine the due date, all things we know don't mean much to begin with).

Even if you choose to have an assisted pregnancy, if you're planning an unassisted birth there are a lot of things you turn down, these being among the first. What it means is that you don't have "concrete evidence" (a phrase I use very loosely here) to confirm or deny a multiple pregnancy, so your imagination runs wild! If morning sickness is worse, or better, if you're larger than normal, or feeling heartburn sooner, or craving something specific, you might be more inclined to think twins. In fact, it's one of the most common things posted about in freebirthing groups online.

Women planning unassisted birth also tend to be more in-tune with energy, their bodies, and intuition. Sometimes, you might feel energetically when your baby has a spiritual companion in the womb, and in that way you might "sense" twins, even if there's only one physical baby gestating.

Another possibility is the phenomenon termed in the medical world as the "disappearing twin," where you conceive twins, but one twin is absorbed into the uterine wall and is "no longer viable." I don't like using those terms, as they seem so medical. I believe that before birth, babies' spirits come and go, and sometimes they decide not to stay and be born. This creates a true "twin energy" in your body, but a twin won't actually manifest.

Of course, there are those times when intuition is crystal clear and dead-on, and twins are present! There are many markers of twins that can be used to determine prenatally, which I won't go over here. Instead, I want to focus on what you can do if this particular intuition comes up for you, and how you can cope in the space of not-knowing.

"Natural" Induction Methods

YOU'VE ENDURED NINE TO ten months of pregnancy. Maybe you're glowing, or maybe you're miserable. Either way, meeting your baby sooner rather than later is an idea almost too tempting to resist.

At this stage in a medically-led pregnancy, around 38-41 weeks, you would be facing an arbitrary deadline of induction for being "overdue." As a freebirther you know that due dates are overused, even abused within the medical model. You might have calculated such a date for yourself, or maybe you chose to let go of the societal expectation to have one and chosen a due month for yourself, or some such thing.

Whichever it is, when you near the end of your pregnancy and you're large and uncomfortable and ready to meet your baby, despite your beliefs about allowing babies to choose their birthdays, you might be tempted to try some "natural" induction methods.

The internet is rife with suggestions, intended for the women facing induction dates by well-meaning but misled care providers. Why do we, as freebirthers, give in to the same imaginary urgency?

We know better, don't we? And yet, we're so conditioned against allowing our bodies and babies to tell us when it's time that we start looking for ways to speed up the process. Simply waiting is just too hard. Waiting is one of the most important things we can learn to do as parents. Waiting for the toddler who is engrossed with a bug on the cement during our walk. Waiting for the preschooler who wants to slide one more time. Waiting for the teenager to do their chores.

Waiting is a critical skill for parents, one that you will use every single day, every single hour, almost. It's a skill that the current "instant gratification" generations already seem deficient in, which makes it that much more important for us to cultivate during pregnancy.

Babies come when they are ready. Bodies birth when they are ready. And even "natural" induction methods can cause harm. There's a time and a place, but in a healthy pregnancy, no interference is needed, even when the pregnancy extends long past the arbitrary due date.

One could argue that "natural induction" is an oxymoronic fallacy in itself. Can one naturally induce something that's not meant to be induced by outside means?

As in everything, freebirthers ought to practice listening to intuition at all times. If you feel inclined to try any induction, ask yourself why. Dig in deep to those feelings. Is this your baby talking? Or your impatience? Is this your body saying it needs a nudge? Or is this your fear of what others think, or of what doctors have said in the past, or some experience another person you know has had?

I had a lot of fear of being "overdue" impressed on me with my first two, both of which went to 41 weeks without medical interference, though I did try "natural" induction methods, including acupressure massage. With my first freebirth, I swore to my baby and myself that I wouldn't do anything extra, natural or not, to force my baby to come early. And boy, did she test me! That pregnancy lasted 42 weeks and 3 days, but in the end I gave birth to a perfectly healthy 9 lb baby. Never once was I afraid or concerned. I was mostly just tired and impatient!

With my most recent freebirth, I was aching. I was exhausted. I had four older kids wearing me out every day, and emotionally I was done. At about 41 weeks, I thought and prayed about what I could do and felt inclined to get a massage. When the therapist offered to add on an "induction package," I felt strongly that it was right. I sent positive thoughts to my baby, telling him this was my way of saying I needed him to come, and that if he was ready, to please come. I also told him if he wasn't ready yet, to not come and I would wait for him. Within 48 hours, I was in labor.

As you know, he was born healthy after an 8 hour labor, weighing more than 10 lbs. He also had a bit of meconium-staining, indicating he had passed meconium in the womb at some point, but he never had any complications from it. I see the situation in hindsight and feel that my intuition was on-point. A little nudge from me benefited my baby, and I'm comfortable with the level of intervention I used at the end of my pregnancy.

My point in all of this is to say that induction is vastly overused in pregnancy, even natural induction. You don't need to do anything to bring your baby safely earth side in most situations. However, if you feel the need to do something, start small and follow these guidelines:

- Only participate in it if you'll enjoy it. Don't force yourself to eat, have sex, or do anything you otherwise wouldn't do. I wouldn't have gone in to see the massage therapist just for an induction massage. I also made sure I was pampering myself and making it enjoyable.
- Stress doesn't help anyone! Don't stress about your "due date," if you picked one. The average pregnancy lasts 41 weeks, but has a recognized variation of 5 weeks! That means it's perfectly normal for some women to birth at 37 weeks, and for others to go to 42 weeks or beyond.
- Don't wear yourself out! Everything in moderation. Don't have a bunch of sex, walk 10 miles, have a marathon meal, and then expect to have anything left for labor should your actions kick it into gear.
- Most food-related methods are more wives' tales, than anything, and the amount you have to eat to have a noticeable effect is ridiculous, to say the least! Eat things you normally eat and not in excess. The stomach ache or bowel changes that could result during labor aren't worth it!
- Avoid Castor Oil, Black Cohosh and Blue Cohosh herbs, and other extreme methods of "natural" induction. Even nature has its dangers, and these are among the worst. Castor oil can cause severe stomach cramping and diarrhea (no one wants that in labor, trust me!). Black and Blue Cohosh can cause severe cramping, problems with bleeding, and risk of infant stroke and heart attack.

Remember, the most guaranteed method of induction is WAITING. Nothing else is as effective or safe, even when you go past 42 weeks. I advocate for using intuition and positive stories to gain understanding and confidence for pregnancy and birth, but the article linked below is one of the best and most comprehensive studies I've found on the subject of due dates and the safety of going "overdue." I highly recommend reading it or using it to help those around you to stop bothering you about your choice to wait.

Placentas and Post-birth Bleeding

AS I MENTIONED AT the beginning of this book, I do not intend for this book to be a one-stop resource for all of the information you need to freebirth. I hope you compile your knowledge from many resources. I can't possibly tell you everything you need to know, but something I have to say may help you some day. Since the birth of the placenta and post-birth bleeding are two extremely common concerns among freebirthers, I would feel remiss not addressing them.

First, I will say that I have never had trouble with bleeding postpartum. In my experiences, my placenta has come in its own time. With my first two births it only took about 20 minutes. With my freebirths it has taken longer, an hour or two. I don't know the reason, but in none of these situations was my bleeding ever a problem. In my freebirths I have gotten settled with my baby, nursed for the first time, made sure my uterus was contracting well (afterbirth pains make it pretty clear, but also press on your uterus to make sure it hardens as it contracts to get your placenta out), and then waited.

Once I feel ready to be separated from my baby, we cut the cord (completely limp and white at this point), and I hand baby off to my husband to weigh and dress. Meanwhile, I squat over a large bowl (sometimes it helps to be in the bathroom), and bear down, tugging just slightly on the umbilical cord. If I feel any resistance, I stop. You can also try blowing into a closed fist, which helps the muscles contract and release.

With my most recent birth, I had a small bit of retained membranes. I could tell because by day nine postpartum, I felt off, almost like I was coming down with something, but I wasn't yet feverish. That day I passed a small string of membranes and felt immediately better. True retained placenta is marked by milk not coming in (because of the hormones from the placenta still inside), fevers, chills, etc. It can turn into a severe septic infection if not passed as soon as possible, and is one of the reasons I would seek assistance postpartum.

Listen to your body and, especially if you have a fever, don't wait to get help. It's inconvenient and possibly even frightening to go to the hospital after having an incredible freebirth, but it's not as inconvenient as the risks involved with waiting.

Associated with the passing of the placenta is postpartum hemorrhage. In the case of excessive bleeding, which is different for everyone, you'll want to watch for feeling faint, light-headed, and generally unwell. If you feel fatigued to the point of not being able to keep your eyes open, or your skin might be cold and clammy to the touch, those are other signs you might have lost too much blood. The amount isn't the important part, it's how you're feeling.

Your cheapest (read: free) option is to cut off a bit of placenta, assuming it's out already, and place it in your cheek. You can swallow if you like, but it's not necessary. Anecdotal evidence suggests that your bleeding could stop within a few minutes with this method. If your placenta isn't out, some say you can use a piece of umbilical cord in its place.

Be aware that the bleeding might come from a tear instead. In this case, you'll want to use a mirror and assess your vulva and vagina and see if you can find where the bleeding is coming from and take action from there.

I've heard numerous stories from freebirthers about placentas taking six, 12, even 24 hours or more to detach and still having positive outcomes. There is no right answer here. Follow your own intuition and trust that you'll know what to do in your unique situation.

There are several supplements and remedies commonly used among freebirthers for placental release, hemorrhage, and easing

afterpains. Use them with caution and wisdom. I feel comfortable recommending the following for your further research:
- Angelica Tincture
- Shepherd's Purse Tincture
- Peppermint Essential Oil
- Afterease Tincture
- Crampbark
- Yunnun Bai Yao (Chinese Herb)

What if I Tear?
Remedies and Recommendations

TAKING A DEEP BREATH, I held the mirror up in front of my vulva.

Red trickled down the delicate folds of skin, showing me the path my baby had taken.

I had torn.

In the wild intensity of labor, consumed with the urge to end the immense pain of uterus contracting and pelvis opening, I pushed with everything I had. Ignoring the potential of the fetal ejection reflex to bring my baby down more gently. I bellowed and thrust my 10 lb baby from my body.

And I tore.

Faced with that reality, I struggled with feelings of confusion and guilt. Should I go to the ER and get stitches? The thought was immediately rejected. It looked like a second degree tear with a large flap of skin hanging down towards my perineum. Could it possibly heal on its own without lasting consequences? I wasn't sure.

Stories of painful sex and bowel or bladder dysfunction lasting months or years after not receiving a timely repair flooded my mind. I did not want my story to be among them.

I sought a blessing from my husband. As Latter-Day Saint Christians (sometimes called Mormons), we believe in the power of prayer and priesthood to heal. The blessing brought me confidence and peace. My intuition pointed me to reach out to some local midwives I thought could be open to coming and assessing my tear.

I texted five of them and went to bed, still feeling restless, open, and vulnerable. I had heard that it's best to have tears repaired sooner rather than later. What if it was too late for mine? Trust, my inner self whispered. I clung to that thought as I drifted off, my hours-old newborn suckling at my breast.

Around midnight one midwife responded. She could come in the morning. Two others couldn't come, but one directed me to a colleague of hers who lived closer to me. I felt a strong surge of trust and hope as I reached out to this midwife, who I didn't know well.

She replied quickly. She could come first thing in the morning and it would cost a third what the other midwife would charge. I immediately felt at ease. This is who I needed to come and advise me.

Her assessment was thorough and professional. She made sure I was comfortable and received my consent to be touched. She was finished so quickly I felt surprised.

"You have a first degree tear." Relief flooded me. Only first degree. That was good. But what about that skin hanging down?

Apparently, the skin had stretched and sheared off in a line, just missing the muscle. The midwife told me I had two choices: I could leave it. It would heal completely, just with "different geography." I liked how she put that. If I wanted to try to get things closer to where they were before, she could put in a few stitches.

Or, she said, we could use seaweed.

I perked up at that. I'd heard that seaweed could repair a tear, but the protocols I found online were vague, at best. This midwife had experience using it with other clients. When you have a skin separation, like I did, the key is to "pack" the seaweed inside the tear, instead of just laying it on top.

She went out and brought back seaweed. A few drops of Frankincense essential oil on the outside of the seaweed makes it adhere to the wound and speed healing, or raw honey can be used. She was gracious enough to apply it for me, inserting the seaweed and holding the flap of skin in place for an entire minute. It BURNED. The healing salt in the seaweed started a fire in my skin. (It's important to note here that you MUST make sure your seaweed is unflavored. Only plain, or salted, should be used.)

She left me with a recipe for Comfrey paste (below) to apply over the top and create a bandage of sorts to help the edges of the tear heal faster. Her instructions were to act as if I had stitches. Keep legs together, stay in bed, avoid scooting on my bottom.

Three days later, while having my first bowel movement, I saw fresh blood on a tissue and thought for sure I'd reopened the tear, but when I looked everything seemed as the midwife had left it - I could still see a bump, or ridge of skin where the flap had been before. It was bleeding, but only a little. After talking with the midwife I felt much better. She explained I probably had just spread my legs a bit far on the toilet and just the edge of the tear had gotten pulled.

I finally got some Comfrey powder to make the paste and applied it. It became sticky as it dried, adhering to my skin and making a protective barrier. It was so effective my bum cheeks got "glued" together at first! It gave me so much mental relief.

At eight weeks postpartum now, I'm pleased to report that everything has healed perfectly. I look different now than before, but there is no dysfunction or pain during sex. I am grateful to that midwife for coming and for sharing her knowledge with me. There is a time and a place for such assistance. If only every woman could have access to such support in pregnancy, birth, and postpartum.

MEDICAL DISCLAIMER: It is fully your responsibility to be knowledgeable about your body and the extent of your own post-birth injuries. The information in this book is intended for information only, and may not be suitable in every scenario. Please seek appropriate medical advice where needed.

Seaweed Protocol

For healing first degree or minor second degree tears

You'll need:

- 1 Sheet of UNFLAVORED Nori Seaweed
- Raw Honey OR Essential Oil such as: Frankincense, Lavender, or Helichrysum
- Scissors
- Handheld mirror
- Clean towel or gauze to clean area
- Chux pad or towel to sit on
- Comfrey paste (recipe below)

Use the bathroom and nurse your baby before beginning. You may want your spouse to help, even if it's just to hold your baby. Sit in a semi-reclined position, legs bent and splayed open. Using the mirror, assess the extent of your tear gently with clean or gloved hands.

Remember the tear could extend up into your vaginal canal, and that there may be multiple small or larger tears.

After using the criteria above to confirm your choice of care, pull out a sheet of seaweed. Cut a piece of seaweed small enough to be tucked INSIDE the tear so any flaps of skin cover it completely and extend just beyond the seaweed, and so the edges of your skin can meet.

Before placing seaweed, dab honey or essential oil of choice on both sides of the seaweed. You may need to use something to dab at blood and clear the skin. Using the mirror, place seaweed inside tear and hold the flap of skin in place for 1 minute or until it remains adhered when you remove pressure.

Using a clean finger, Popsicle stick, or spoon, apply a small amount of Comfrey paste to the outside of the tear. Let it sit for a moment. It will not dry or harden, but it will set a bit.

You can let your bottom air out or put an adult diaper or pad and underwear on at this point. You may find the Comfrey paste makes your labia or bum cheeks stick together a bit. If this happens, recline and use your mirror to pull the skin apart gently without pulling the tear apart. Follow a "mermaid protocol" and keep your legs together as much as possible the first five days. Don't scoot your bottom, as this can pull on it as well, and shuffle when you walk. Avoid stairs and don't drive. Success of the Seaweed Protocol depends on following these instructions closely and correctly identifying your tear as first degree or minor second degree.

If the seaweed falls out because the tear reopens, repeat (this shouldn't happen if this process is done correctly and within 24 hours of giving birth).

You can still use a peri bottle or sitz bath, even take a bath, after applying the Seaweed Protocol.

The seaweed will be used by your skin to nourish the area as it heals, and it should dissolve completely.

No flap of skin? The Seaweed Protocol can be used as a bandage of sorts on a surface tear, although it will need to be replaced more often.

Comfrey Paste

You will need:
- 3 Tablespoons Comfrey Root Powder
- 2 teaspoons Raw Honey (can use Manuka Honey, if desired)
- Wheat germ oil (or olive, avocado, or other healing oil)

Method:

Mix first two ingredients together, warming honey if needed. Slowly mix in oil until it is a spreadable consistency but not runny. It should look similar to your newborn's meconium poop. Add more honey to thicken if needed. Store in airtight container for up to one week.

The Wisdom found in Not-Knowing

WHAT DO YOU HAVE when you don't have "knowledge" as it would be defined in scientific circles? You have intuition, which could also be called wisdom, and when combined with a willingness to let go of the outcome, this is a powerful type of understanding to cultivate. It will serve you time and time again in your pregnancy, birth, and parenting.

Letting go isn't particularly simple, however. Our minds tend to latch onto ideas and obsess over them, whether they're positive or negative, and this obsession can be harmful when taken to extremes. My particular challenge this past month has been to let go of when my baby is coming. At the time of this writing, I'm almost 39 weeks pregnant by my best estimated due date.

Around 34 weeks I started obsessing over whether this baby would come early. All of my babies are more typically "late" (though I'm sure we all know by now that "late" is a silly, irrelevant label created by the medical model of birth). I thought maybe by Christmas, because wouldn't that be fun? But no. I thought New Year's, but no. As these significant dates have passed, I've finally begun to let go of the "maybe" and focus more on being present, enjoying this pregnancy, and nesting in our new home, as we have just moved.

Obsessing only made it harder for me to cope with the other stressors I was experiencing (the physical fatigue and mental load of moving, for one). It made it hard for me to fully enjoy the holiday with family, especially with everyone giving me a wide-eyed look and exclaiming that surely I couldn't have THAT much time left. Every encounter left me exhausted, and even my husband picked up the habit, though I finally communicated to him that it wasn't helpful to have him eyeing my belly as if it would pop suddenly!

I've entered a waiting time where most pregnant women go at this stage. It's made much easier by my willingness to let go and let this baby be born on a day of his choice.

So it is with the twin-feeling. It will go away eventually or be confirmed/denied by some obvious sign. For some that will be ultrasound, if that's something you subscribe to. For others that will be hearing the heartbeat and only finding one, using either fetoscope or doppler. And still others, perhaps the most patient of us all, will sit with not-knowing until labor begins and mother nature herself determines twins or not.

Whatever your path, the best and healthiest thing you can do for yourself is to relax and let go. If research will help you come to that place, then by all means learn the symptoms for twins and try to determine for yourself if there's a second baby present. Or plan a mid-pregnancy ultrasound, if the benefits of that peace of mind would outweigh the risks for you. But know this: at some point in your pregnancy, you will again be confronted with the same lesson to learn, the wisdom in letting go.

Considering Ultrasound

There are others who speak much more eloquently on this subject, such as in the podcast recommended above, so my little piece to add is just this: Whether or not to receive an ultrasound during your pregnancy is your choice. In my opinion, ultrasound can be a valuable tool, but it all depends on your perspective and what you would do with the information an ultrasound provides. For me, ultrasound offers a snapshot into my womb where I can see that the placenta is growing up out of the way, and my baby is fully formed and healthy. I choose ultrasound because I would want to know if these things weren't the case, and my birthing choices would probably change if the situation were different.

This isn't the case for all women who choose freebirth. Many feel that ultrasounds cause too much harm for any benefit they might bring. Harm that, for the most part, goes unrecognized in the medical industry. I've included a number of podcasts and articles in this section for you to peruse on your own. Weigh the evidence, read the opinions, but at the end of the day follow your faith, not your fear.

My friends and family members get pregnant and show off ultrasound photos or videos after nearly every appointment, even with healthy, normal pregnancies. Sometimes I'm a little jealous that they get to "see" their baby so often, but then I remember that I'm doing what *I* feel is right for my baby, and there are other ways to connect. If you don't want an ultrasound but desire a stronger connection with your unborn baby, try the following:

- Talk to your baby.
- Choose or compose a special song just for this baby and play/sing it often.
- Try your hand at birth art, in any medium.
- Prepare for the birth - buy supplies, choose and decorate your ideal birthing space, buy some clothes (or wash and fold hand-me-downs.)
- Meditate, pray, or visualize.
- Listen to baby's heartbeat with a fetoscope, measure your fundal height, or create some sort of daily, weekly, or monthly ceremony or habit (like a prenatal visit!) meant to draw you closer to your baby.

This is a very short list, and there are many things you could do to create a bond before your baby arrives. The important thing is that you don't feel left out of connecting with your baby.

"That's all well and good for me," you might say, "But my family is driving me nuts/is offended/etc." I get it. It's hard not to feel the social pressure when your Pinterest and Facebook feeds are filled with everyone else throwing picture-perfect gender reveal parties. And especially if it's your first, everyone wants to celebrate with you.

Good intentions all around, but this is critical for you to remember now: this is not their pregnancy, their baby, or their birth that YOU are preparing for. If you're uncomfortable with ultrasounds, do not get one just to please your mother-in-law or put your friend's mind at ease. Instead, stand firm in your decision and consider trying one of the following to help your family and friends still feel involved in the pregnancy:

- Have a baby shower (let someone else plan it, like that mother-in-law mentioned previously)
- Have a Mother Blessing Ceremony - this is for you, so make sure you let a trusted friend plan it and be highly involved with how you want it to go. Celebrate your pregnancy, pamper yourself and your friends, and only invite those who can truly be positive. It's a great idea to do a group fear release during a gathering like this.
- Invite them to your birth - obviously only if they will be a beneficial energy and help. Never invite anyone to your birth, freebirth or otherwise, who would disrupt the atmosphere with their own fears or opinions.
- Go baby gear shopping with them.
- Prepare postpartum freezer meals with them.

There are times when the toxicity from a family member or friend is too much to even consider inviting them to something. In those cases, never feel obligated to invite them. Even if your intention is to help those around you be more involved, you shouldn't sacrifice your own mental well-being to entertain anyone. So, all of this is optional and should be done in the spirit of love on all sides.

Finding Intuition

"Sometimes the bravest thing you can do is listen to the soft whisper in your heart telling you which way to go."

- The Better Man Project

YOU'LL HEAR THIS A lot in freebirth circles, especially. "What does your intuition say?" "Follow your intuition."

But what does it mean to "follow" intuition? How do you learn to listen to intuition in the first place? And what do you do when it feels like you don't have any intuition?

First off, understand that everyone around you, even those you most admire for their ability to tune in to that innate part of themselves and follow through on what they seem to know to be true, everyone is still learning about their own intuition and how to follow it. It's a lifelong part of this mortal existence. It is a skill you can hone and improve upon.

What is Intuition?

Intuition is the reason I recommend researching stories rather than studies. Studies are full of reasoning that may or may not have any implications for your situation, no matter how much you 'fit the mold' for a condition or situation described by the medical model. You can read as many studies as you like, discovering all of the risk percentages and how likely something is to occur, but be wary. Those numbers can be hard to drown out when your intuition says to go one way and the numbers say that way is dangerous or irresponsible.

There are a host of things that most medical providers will tell you contain too much risk. Most hospitals, doctors, nurses, even many midwives, run their entire practice and base all of their policies on preventing any "statistically significant" risk. That means that even if the risk is only 1 in a 1000, or 1 in 10,000, often times they will tell you it's too dangerous, that your baby could be harmed or die, and they will recommend oftentimes extreme treatment despite higher rates of problems occurring from said treatment.

"Studies" done about these things will often show numbers that don't make sense. For instance, I've read a few studies that indicate there is no heightened rate of cesarean section associated with induction prior to 40 weeks. In fact, some of these studies, even large ones, seem to indicate the opposite you would expect: that early induction at around 39 weeks improves outcomes for babies.

Maybe it does. But after reading thousands of stories from women who were induced and forced into cesarean sections due to the famous "cascade of interventions," I have to believe that there is an inherent and invisible bias present in these studies. Often they're done as part of hospital programs that implement certain policies to reduce cesarean sections specifically, so of course providers will act differently during the induction process than they would otherwise. In these instances, it isn't the induction at 39 weeks lowering the cesarean section rate; it's the new policies that are put into place increasing providers' awareness and willingness to wait.

Waiting is the number one under-utilized option in a medical setting. They're too afraid to wait. They're too afraid to listen to your intuition. And it's incredibly difficult to listen to your intuition in the hospital, especially. Monitors blinking numbers, strangers spouting opinions dressed as facts, all with an authority that most people, most women, perceive as greater than their own.

When you freebirth, you have to accept that you have the greatest authority in the room, aside from God. You walk with Him to bring this child into the world, and no one else is equal with you in that situation. No one you invite into your space, no one you hire. You bring people into your space for their knowledge, the wisdom of their experience, or their ability to comfort and assist you. You do not bring them into your space for their fear, and in fact, you should be prepared to ask anyone to leave when they start to communicate fear in your birth space.

How to Discern Intuition in the Face of Fear

I can't tell you exactly how to discern your own intuition. It most likely feels and acts differently for you than for me. Just based on my experience talking with my husband, he and I interpret intuition very differently. For me it comes immediately through a feeling when I consider a matter. For my husband it more often comes in a subtle way, after much inner thought and pondering. My intuition is served well by gathering outside information in the form of conversations with others, books, internet, and other media. My husband's intuition is better served by less outside searching, more inward thinking.

It could be different for you. Pursue your own revelations in whatever way feels natural to you. And if you try something and feel more confused, more uncertain, then take a step back and focus internally. Perhaps what you need isn't out there, it's inside of you.

We often search outside ourselves when we feel uncertain. We look for something to grasp hold of, some authority we can depend on that isn't our own, that we trust more. Therefore, cultivating trust in yourself is a key part of listening to and acting on your intuition. It's wise to study different aspects of pregnancy, birth, and postpartum in preparation for your freebirth. It's well and good to ask others for their opinion. Do not, however, allow these facts or opinions to take the place of your own thoughts and feelings. Your intuition will serve you better the more you follow it. It weakens when you ignore it.

You won't always feel an absence of fear when you have intuition, but it's a good rule of thumb that you shouldn't act based on fear itself. Try to find a place of peace or relative calm before proceeding, even in an emergent situation. This will be easier in pregnancy, in general, than it is during labor. Contractions are often all-consuming, and pain takes us into a more primal, instinctive part of ourselves, which simultaneously makes it easier and harder to access intuition. If you can take a breath, wait for the contraction and immediate surge of emotion to pass, close your eyes and feel into yourself with a prayer for the ability to discern, then you will know what your intuition is telling you. Then your job is to act on that intuition, even if it doesn't make sense, even if it isn't necessarily taking you where you wanted to go.

Trust yourself. Trust God. Develop your intuition, and you will have the experience you are meant to have with this birth.

BOOK: "Mother's Intention: How Belief Shapes Birth" by Kim Wildner and Chelsea Wildner

When Fear Comes to Your Birth

"The fear will never go away as long as you continue to grow. If you are waiting for fear to go away before you take any chances, you have the wrong idea. As long as you are stretching your responsibilities, fear is inevitable."

- Dr. Susan Jeffers, author of "Feel the Fear and Do it Anyway"

Fear shows up in some form at most births. It's part of nearly every birth story I've ever read. What that should tell you is, first, that it is normal to experience fear in birth. It is our conscious, evolved brain's way of telling us something overwhelmingly powerful is happening, and those sensations translate into fear under the instinctual pretense of keeping us alive. When we feel pain or other overwhelming physical sensations, our bodies send signals through hormones and nerves and energy channels, sometimes translating into coherent thoughts such as, "I can't do this," "I'm going to die," "I'm not big enough," "I'm ripping apart," etc. In addition to thoughts, these physical messages can come across as raw, pure, inexplicable emotion.

There are dozens of birthing courses and mentorships available online and in-person focusing on helping women overcome fear in childbirth. There's this belief that seems to circle like a dark clouds over the heads of pregnant women: fear is BAD. Fear will sabotage your birth. Fear will make you have a cesarean section or other trauma. Fear is the root of it all.

The truth is, fear is helpful, normal, and can even be beneficial. That's not to say we ignore our fear and do nothing when we experience it. What that means is that fear comes to us to highlight the darkened areas of our minds, to reveal missing or incorrect truths, to teach us and, ultimately, to help us grow. Feeling fear during your birth doesn't mean you fail to have an empowered, autonomous birth. We are capable of working through that fear in the moment and passing through it to whatever end that experience has in store.

It's false to say that all cesarean sections and traumatic or medical assistance births are caused by fear or false beliefs. Some babies are meant to come that way. Remember, they are individual beings with lessons to learn too. Those lessons begin the moment they enter their mortal bodies, which I believe happens intermittently during pregnancy, and then more permanently during the birth process (although it seems that some babies never quite enter their bodies fully, and these babies don't stay very long, either).

PODCAST: How to Deal with Fear in Pregnancy

No woman fails who feels fear in her births. I've spent more than six years taking classes, meditating, using Hypnosis for childbirth, attending conferences and workshops to learn how to eliminate fear. Having the powerful experience of going through five pregnancies and births in less than seven years, preparing for each, carefully paying attention to any fear that comes up or might come up, I've gone into labor each time and still found fear waiting for me in transition.

With my first three births I wondered what I had done wrong, or where I had neglected to eliminate fear. After my fourth birth, a super fast three-hour birth that left me doubting I wanted to go through this again, I began to catch a glimmer of understanding. My motivation to avoid fear had brought me immense growth through the study and practices I implemented during each pregnancy, leading to wonderful, though "imperfect" birth experiences.

With my fifth pregnancy, I felt alarmed as I realized that I had read nearly everything available about eliminating fear and inviting pleasure in birth. So many books, articles, courses, everything.

When you give birth in rapid succession to a number of babies, opportunities for the resource pool of information to refresh are limited. Simply, not enough time had passed since my last pregnancy for much new information to come to light. My research-oriented self was stumped. How could I improve, how could I eliminate those last shreds of fear, if there was nothing new to try?

The answer, for me, was to just be. Be with this pregnancy, be with this birth. Find within myself the intuition and wisdom I needed, and stop seeking it outside myself in any form. I still browsed online, but I tried not to get attached to finding "the answer," and instead noticed more deeply what was happening within myself as the weeks turned into months, flutters turned into kicks, and my fifth baby revealed the gift of wisdom he would give me: Deeper intuition, deeper trust, and a more complete understanding of fear and the role it plays in birth.

> "Everything you want is on the other side of fear…if you can learn to derail [fear] when it comes,
>
> your definition of what is possible will start changing."
>
> - Michael Laronn

FACING THE FEAR OF OTHERS

Your partner will likely be the first to know your plans to freebirth, if you have a partner. But after that, who should you tell and how can you be certain that they will respond positively?

The fact is, who you tell should be dependent on who you trust, and you must let go of the idea that you have much influence on how they react.

The majority of people, especially in the American culture, will show and speak fear and uncertainty when you mention plans to birth at home, much less without an attendant. They may become critical and confrontational, or attempt to persuade and manipulate. This is why I recommend you only tell those who are truly supportive of you and those who will be at your birth. Even so, you may find that someone you thought would respond well doesn't, and your plans for who attends your birth may need to shift to exclude anyone with a deeply negative mindset.

People tend to assume that when your choices are different than theirs, it means their choices are somehow invalid or under attack. Especially those in a victim mindset will take everything personally.

The trick is to not take their response personally, which can be difficult when it's family, a close friend, or someone you see every day.

"The questioning many of us are doing about the system, about birth, about autonomy is NECESSARY. And it's not a commentary on people or births or scenarios where people chose NOT to question. My choices are not a commentary on your lack of choice, your poor choice or just your different choice." - Maryn Green, Indie Birth Association

How to Respond

Most responses you get will fall into one of two camps: the Fearful and the Awed. The Fearful camp is much larger, of course, and responses from someone in this group include things like the following:

- What if something goes wrong?
- If I hadn't been in the hospital, had a cesarean, etc. my baby would have died.
- Isn't that illegal?
- You're going to kill your baby/ yourself.
- Example from a relative or friend about everything that could go wrong.

How you respond will vary depending on your willingness to engage, and perhaps the tone of the individual you're talking to, or

how well you know them. A great way to diffuse a fearful naysayer is to start by validating their fears:
- "You're right, rarely there are complications that require intervention."
- "There's a small chance something could go wrong."
- "Everyone has a different body/experience."
- "Sometimes babies or mothers do die in birth."
- "Those situations are extremely rare, and I trust myself to know when to go to the hospital or see a doctor."

People expect you to argue, or get flustered and upset. They don't expect you to say that they are right. What they are saying is true, at least on some level. You can validate that and often diffuse a combative individual without further argument. If they continue to attack your choice, hold your hand up and set this boundary: "I won't discuss this with you until you do more research (or until you're calmer, more respectful, etc.)"

Change the subject or walk away. You can come back to this boundary as often as needed, and make it personal to you.

Another great response. which I learned from Maryn and Margo with the Indie Birth Association, is to start with the words "Well, actually…." and a statement of truth. This could look like the following:
- "Well, actually, those high risk situations are rare and are most often detected by obvious symptoms well before it becomes a true emergency."
- "Well, actually, many emergencies are created by the policies and procedures/interventions in the hospital that prevent birth unfolding naturally and safely."
- "Well, actually, birth at home is perfectly legal."
- "Well, actually, birth at home is very safe for low risk women."

And then you can, if you choose, immediately follow that with more detail, delivered in confidence. Your goal in these encounters shouldn't be to change their opinion or give them a thorough education on the subject. Focus instead on planting a seed. If at any point you feel burdened by answering questions or deflecting attacks, go back to your boundary, set it firmly and stick to it.

It's always an option to set your boundary from the beginning of the conversation and refuse to engage. If they can't respect that, you certainly don't owe them any insight into your private life or personal decisions.

A faction of the "Fearful" camp is a group of individuals I term "Fearful and Hostile." These individuals typically strive to assert authority or control over you and your choices by becoming aggressive or threatening. Physical aggression is never acceptable and should be reported as abuse or harassment through the proper channels.

Emotional abuse, while sometimes difficult to detect, is just as damaging and may require some form of separation from the individual in your life. This could look like temporarily walking out of the room and taking a break from the conversation, or taking permanent action towards breakup, divorce (in the case of a spouse), or no contact at all during your pregnancy.

Not every interaction or relationship will be so extreme or require such drastic action. So what do you do when someone is hostile towards your choice to freebirth, but you want to do your best to preserve the relationship?

As long as you aren't in physical danger, the first thing to do is establish your boundary, make the other person aware of it, and ask if they can agree to respect it. Sometimes these individuals might threaten you or your plans for freebirth. Here are some things you can say to those who tell you that home birth is illegal, or if they threaten to call police, CPS, or other authorities:

- I have the legal right to give birth at home. In most countries this is a lesser-known reality. home birth is legal in all 50 states in the U.S., whether midwifery is legal or not. If you live in another country, be sure to check your local laws regarding birth.
- I have done my research and studied the risks; this is the safest / best choice for me and my baby. This statement can be followed by asking the other person to do their research before discussing it with you again. Feel free to give them resources to start with, but don't do the research for them. Do set a boundary for yourself that if they choose to only engage in fear-based conversation without learning more about the subject, then you will not discuss your pregnancy or birth with them.
- This is MY choice to make. With the often patriarchal views of our society, a woman's right to choose in pregnancy and birth is rarely recognized or honored. Remind others that this is your

body, your baby, your choice. In the case of birth partners, such as your husband or the baby's father, it is important to remind him that although he helped make the baby, decisions about the place and with whom you give birth affect your body, not his. In the end, he needs to respect your authority in birthing the child you created together.

- Uninvite them from your birth, or don't invite them in the first place. I go into more detail about when and how to do this in chapter x, but it bears repeating: everyone at your birth should be 100% supportive of your choice to birth unassisted. It is better to cause a little offense before the birth than have huge regrets afterward if the person shows up and sabotages your experience by calling 911 or spouting their fears in your space during a vulnerable time.

The second camp I mentioned earlier is the easiest to interact with. Those in the "Awe" category will usually say something like the following, although watch for their words to be mixed with or followed by fear:

- Wow! All by yourself? I wish I were brave enough to do that!
- I always wanted to birth at home.
- I could never do that!
- Further praise, statements of admiration or disbelief (but not critical).

These individuals will often ask questions about how you had a freebirth or plan to do it, and what you plan to do in certain situations (such as baby not breathing, postpartum hemorrhage, etc.) These questions shouldn't be responded to with offense. In fact, these are the questions most worth your time to answer, because your knowledge and confidence will lead people in awe of your decisions to assimilate the normalcy and safety of birth, even to the point of defending you to others within your social circle or family because they admire your confidence.

They might never choose to freebirth themselves, but they will maintain respect for your choices.

WHAT TO DO WHEN SOMEONE CALLS 911

Not everyone has the intuition and faith in your body, your baby, and birth that you do. And most people have a lot of fear surrounding birth. When fear overwhelms, sometimes even a trusted friend, family member, or traditional birth attendant will call for emergency services without consulting with you first, or ignoring your insistence that everything is fine and that you don't need any medical assistance.

So, first thing, make sure those that attend your birth understand that you'll tell them if you need more help, and make sure they trust you. There's nothing worse than having someone who doesn't trust you at your birth!

Second, stay calm and rock your birth, mama! In laborland, it's difficult to reason and make logical decisions, which is why it's so important to make sure everyone at your birth is 100% aware and supportive of your decision to freebirth. You can't always control how someone will react in the midst of labor. You have a few choices in how to react.

Emergency personnel have two goals when they arrive: make sure you're stable and get you to the hospital. You can refuse anything you don't want, including giving them access to your home, birth space, or body. Whomever called 911 may invite them in, but you can refuse their care. You could also allow them to check you out, if only to give others peace of mind (though that's not your job). Ultimately, you'll need to decide whether to transfer to the hospital, let emergency personnel stay but refuse to transfer, or refuse to transfer and ask them to leave.

Regardless of what anyone says, you are in control here, and you get to decide when, or if, you go to the hospital. If you decide to stay home, consider the atmosphere you're now birthing in. Unless the person who called is also asked to leave, you may find them hostile, fearful, or openly anxious if emergency personnel leave. How will you navigate that while in labor?

Very rarely, police may be the first to respond, and they're less likely to know what to do and more likely to make frightening statements or threats out of fear. Know your rights. Be calm as you can be.

The best option is, of course, to prevent this situation by having full communication with everyone invited to your birth beforehand, including telling them which situations would necessitate a call for an ambulance. Don't let your own fear over how they'll react to your freebirth plans sabotage your birth experience. Move forward with confidence, even in the face of fear, whether yours or anyone else's.

When Birth Ends with Death

"In the end we'll all become stories."
- *Margaret Atwood*

RECENTLY, A STORY CIRCULATED around Facebook and the news where a planned freebirth turned into a tragedy. The story isn't mine to tell, so suffice it to say the mother's water was broken for several days and reportedly meconium-stained. When she asked in a group online, she was told by some to seek assistance, and by many others to not worry. She eventually went in to the hospital after her baby stopped moving. Unfortunately, she found out her baby had died, and she birthed her stillborn baby with assistance.

Afterward, the mother said she was at peace with every decision she had made during her labor. The internet, of course, raged. This grieving mother received death threats. Her story was used as propaganda by those who oppose home birth and especially freebirth. And the online freebirth support community where she shared her original post during labor was shut down due to internet trolls sending further death threats to the creator.

None of us want to consider death as a possible outcome of our pregnancy or birth, but not being willing to face and accept it is exactly why birth in the U.S. is in the state it's in. We live in a society that blames the victim. When death happens, even of natural causes, everyone questions "Was it necessary? Could I (or someone else) have done more to prevent it?"

We seem to not know how to process death in healthy ways. This leads to a dramatic fear of death, despite its inevitability, and drastic actions are taken to prevent it, even paying the price of quality of life in order to achieve quantity of life.

Among women preparing to freebirth, I see three typical attitudes: rejection of the possibility (including refusal to consider or prepare for it); willingness to prepare, seek knowledge about when assistance "should" be sought to avoid it (sometimes with fear, other times with peace); last, an acceptance so absolute the woman is prepared to freebirth at home despite, perhaps, knowing about a complication that could increase risk of, or result in, death. This last woman is often resolute in her opinion that even if something could be done to prolong or possibly save her baby's life, she would rather her baby live it's only moments at home in her arms, surrounded by love rather than in a hospital surrounded by medical equipment.

There is no right view, no correct path for everyone, just as there is no one path to take for pregnancy and birth.

The one thing we should never do is project our path onto someone else's story. Offer love, hope, empathy. Bring meals, or serve where possible when it happens locally. Defend the mother's right to decide for her child, and don't join the naysayers that shame the victim for not doing more. She's already in mourning; she deserves comfort, not death threats.

The reality is that some babies die. In the United States, even with a high rate of hospital births, our infant and maternal mortality rates are shameful. If hospitals and medically-assisted birth were the cure, we would have the lowest rates in the world. But we don't. We have among the highest. Many doctors, nurses, and "medwives" disregard and disrespect women out of fear of death and the legal liability that comes with it in a society that fears it. The change doesn't begin with policies. The change needs to begin within us, the women giving birth.

Death is part of life. By embracing it we embrace life more fully than otherwise possible. Striving to reach a place in your soul where you can be unafraid of death will allow you to access your intuition in ways you've never known before. You will know when to stay home and when to seek assistance, because when the moment comes to decide you will not be afraid, rather you will feel peace and power in your choice. This is what autonomous birth is about: being in a space to make ANY choice you need to, without being swayed by outside opinions and fears. Whether you birth at home by yourself or choose assistance, you need to be able to look inside yourself and say, "I am not afraid," in the face of anything that might happen during pregnancy, labor, or birth.

You will know if unassisted birth is right because you will not be afraid.

You will know having a self-led pregnancy is right because you will not be afraid.

You will also know when hiring a midwife is right, or seeing a doctor, or going into the emergency room in labor, or saying "yes" to a medication, intervention, or even a cesarean section is right because deep down YOU WILL NOT BE AFRAID.

There may be feelings similar to fear because of the uncertainty surrounding what you are about to experience, especially if you've never been through it before. But this is not fear. This is curiosity's cousin, anxiety, and it's healthy in small doses. It keeps us alert, alive, questioning.

My personal belief is that preparation and knowledge, when coupled with faith and hope, are the best ways to combat fears. This looks different for everyone, but if you find that you fear death or any negative outcome in regards to pregnancy or birth or even postpartum and parenting, search yourself for these things. Do you simply need more knowledge? Do you need to prepare in some way? Do you need to increase in faith or establish hope?

Act on those intuitive promptings, and move forward knowing that you will always have everything you need within.

Freebirth Stories

All of the following stories and photos are shared with permission from the women they belong to.

"I like stories where women save themselves."
— *Neil Gaiman, "The Sleeper and the Spindle"*

The Birth of Juniper Jane Clinger
Submitted by Anonymous

JUNIPER JANE WAS A surprise to all. When we moved to Ukraine, we had no intention of making any more babies from scratch, ever. We had hoped that we'd find a baby here, that we'd bring home a child or two, and I had hoped specifically for a baby girl. At the end of our first summer here, spent mostly out of doors in fresh air and enjoying good food with good company, a miscalculation in timing occurred and in that moment I knew that we'd just invited a new spirit to join our family. Two weeks later we received confirmation that the invitation had been received and accepted.

I don't normally experience terrible morning sickness, and it usually starts around 8 weeks and lasts for about 15 weeks. My nausea started almost right away, and lasted a full 18 weeks. I was as active as I could tolerate, but found myself drawn to the dark quiet of my room often. I was able to put on a happy face, stay active in church, and even endured many very crowded, very hot public transportation rides without actually getting physically ill, which will be a badge of pride I wear for life.

Just as the nausea was passing, and I expected to enter the easy second trimester, my body decided to go into hormone producing hyperdrive. My hips spread and symptoms of SPD began to appear. The feeling that my hips might drop my legs at any moment, coupled with a piercing lower back pain kept me from being as active as I would normally have been during this stage of pregnancy. It also began to affect my mood, making me feel useless, defeated, and just plain down. At about 20-22 weeks though, on Christmas Eve, we discovered that the baby I was carrying was not going to be a John Gabriel Clinger, but was in fact a little mystery girl Clinger. We were so surprised, and so happy, even though we would have been perfectly happy with another baby boy additon.

Having attended my sister Holly's last birth, in Peru a little more than a year before, I was wary to have a hospital birth experience here. I am wary of hospital birth in general, having had three of them, and then having Daniel at home five years ago. The only problem was, NO ONE has their babies at home here. Not in the countryside, not on accident, and definitely not on purpose. We made our intentions clear to the American Medical Center, and while they thought we were crazy, nobody told us not to, so we made arrangements to have a friend of ours, a retired midwife, come stay for the last few weeks of pregnancy and help us catch this baby at home.

We invested in some simple monitoring tools and for the most part, I kept track of all my vitals on my own. Everything progressed normally and healthfully. There was just the pain from the SPD, and then eventually sciatica that was bothering me. It got so bad, that sweeping the floor would send my back into spasms and make me feel like I might collapse. At one point, I got out of bed too quickly and tried to walk too immediately and I did collapse. That taught me that I needed to go slower and let my body realign every time I switched from sitting or lying down, to a standing position. Of course, my nesting manifested itself through my obsession with having clean floors, so every day I proceeded to torture my body, to satiate my mind.

Because of the abundance of ripening and softening hormones in my body, I began to feel like this baby would try to make her appearance early. Even though I'd progressively carried each of my babies longer with each pregnancy, my head kept worrying that something would go wrong, or would be different this time, and she would try to come too early, or something would go wrong. Every time I would pray about it though I would get the comforting confirmation that she was going to be perfect, and everything was going to work out as it should. Because of my anxiety, I did have my husband, Karl, give me a few priesthood blessings throughout the pregnancy, just to help ease my mind, and that really did help. Even with these confirmations though, I felt so much joy when I'd reach a new milestone.

At 25 weeks I was relieved that she was now considered viable, even if she might have a tough time of it. At 30 weeks I was excited that she was not only viable, but that she'd probably spend much less time in the hospital if she was born then. Then each week after that became a little celebration within myself that we'd made it another week and she was getting bigger and stronger and healthier every day.

At 35 weeks I finally began to relax. I'd had babies at 35 weeks and they were tiny but healthy. It was about this time though that I began to have doubts about bringing our midwife to us. I was wondering if we'd planned the right timing. I was worried about housing, which isn't generally a big deal, but again, I was having some elevated levels of anxiety with this pregnancy and the thought of bringing her here began to be more stressful than the idea of having no one here to help. I talked to her about it not feeling quite right, and wasn't entirely truthful about our plans to proceed with having the baby at home. We did continue to have open lines of communication with the American Medical Clinic, but wanted to use them only in case of emergency.

It's an interesting process, planning on having a baby without a professional birth attendant present. I have a deep respect for the opinions of professionals on having unassisted births. As I researched all the possible outcomes, and listened in on conversation threads in Midwife groups, I began to learn the things that scare midwives. The more I learned, the more birth seems to be a miracle. It's not about trusting or not trusting women's bodies, or the process when midwives talk about "knowing too much." It's really that sometimes things do happen, and sometimes they happen so infrequently that you're caught unaware, but hopefully not unprepared. It seemed the more I learned, and the more I tried to prepare, I realized how much time and experience I would actually need in order to ACTUALLY be prepared.

So, I focused on the two main concerns: bleeding, and breathing and I taught all the different methods to Karl as I learned them myself. We also acquired several natural remedies to stop bleeding, and Karl, my husband, brushed up on his resuscitation skills. We also had the priesthood with us. I knew Karl would do everything in his power, and within God's plan to make sure we were fine. This was not a decision we came to easily, or took lightly, and we included our Heavenly Father in the process, or more accurately, we relied on Him throughout.

Then, as 37 weeks approached I began to feel silly that I'd even worried about her being too early. I was caught in that trap of being physically done and not mentally prepared to have a baby. I began to fear in new ways. I wasn't ready for another child to care for. I was done with diapers, and breastfeeding, and long nights. My youngest had just turned five and is teaching himself how to read and write, and has engaging conversations with me! This wasn't in my plan. And then there was guilt for feeling all these things. I also was feeling the pain and the trauma associated with having been left nearly alone to take care of Daniel, as Karl was in the middle of his traveling work-years. I didn't want to do it all again, all alone. He's always been so very busy around the times we have had had babies, with no ability to stay home when I needed him, or to stay up at night if I needed him. I was afraid of being alone again, and most surprising to me, I was afraid of the pain of labor I knew I would have to endure.

Even though I'd done it three times without medication, and I'd even looked forward to it a few of those times, I was not looking forward to it this time. I knew it was hard work. I knew that it was doable, but I also knew that once it starts there's no end until you feel like your whole body has come apart to allow entrance into this world, and that was intimidating to me this time.

I skipped church the last two weeks. My belly had grown immense, my back was sore no matter what I did, and I had no ability to put a smile on my face if I didn't feel like smiling and didn't want to answer questions about when, or where, or if I was ready. Honestly, how do you even answer those questions? Who really knows when? Is anyone really and truly ready for this?

At 38 weeks and three days, our fabulous Mission President's wife, and Sister Plaster, our couples' missionary made our family dinner and brought it to the house. I had been contracting somewhat regularly for about a week at this time, on and off, but it would always stop at some point. Birth felt imminent though, and their food was just what I think I needed to push me over the edge into readiness. Homemade beef stew, a huge fresh green salad, fresh baked dinner rolls, oatmeal cookies, and cinnamon rolls for breakfast the next day. We wolfed it down, watched a movie together as a family (Star Wars: The Phantom Menace, as it was May the 4th) and slept contently that night.

I woke up just after five in the morning on May 5th to a couple of contractions that finally felt like they were the kind that work. I continued to have them, throughout the morning, even though they were not terribly consistent. I even timed them for a while and they were anywhere from ten to twenty minutes apart. They felt like real contractions, but they weren't lasting a full minute yet, and they were still so inconsistently timed. I felt, nonetheless, that this was labor and I prepared our room and the bathroom for the possibility of birth.

I made our bed up with a plastic sheet and made sure there were gloves, trash bags, and chux pads easily accessible in either room. I ate my allotted cinnamon rolls for breakfast. I think I had something else too, but I can't remember. Karl is good at keeping me fed. I put on Harry Potter and the Half-Blood Prince and napped a bit. During the nap, they spaced out to about 20-30 minutes apart. Karl had an appointment scheduled that day at 1:00 p.m. and so I was paying attention to whether or not it seemed like a good idea for him to go. At noon, things were still spaced out and I gave him the thumbs up to go ahead. I'd message him if things changed.

While he was gone I watched a few episodes of a show I've been watching on Netflix, and timed contractions. They ranged from 4 to 8 minutes apart, and were lasting about a minute, but still under a minute sometimes. I wasn't concerned by this, but a little disappointed that they weren't more regular. I ate leftovers from the night before and decided to lay down and take another little nap. They spaced out again to about twenty minutes apart. I was just waking up from my nap when Karl got home. We have wind chimes over the door, so I can always hear when he gets home. As I laid there with my eyes closed coming out of my sleep, I had a huge double peaked contraction. He'd brought me an ice cream sandwich, which I gladly ate, but knew that would likely be the last thing I ate before she was born. That was just after four o'clock in the afternoon.

I had the kids start some potatoes baking, so that they'd have something to eat whenever they got hungry. I also took several drops of Willow flower essence, by Bachs flower essences. I had been feeling a lot of anxiety over the pain of labor. I wasn't afraid from a health concern point of view, just afraid of the pain itself. I've always hoped for a painless labor and easy breezy transition, but so far it just hasn't been in the cards for me.

I cope well enough, I definitely survive it well, but it still hurts like the dickens, and I just simply didn't want to go through it. Willow flower is supposed to help you face your fears, and I had been adding it to my water for the past several days to help with that. I know from experience, that the less afraid you are of contractions the easier it is to cope with them. From that point forward, I contracted about every four minutes, consistently, and personally, I think the Willow helped quite a bit.

I remember feeling a bit restless, and Karl went and filled up the bathtub, just in case I wanted to labor in it. It's a deep tub, but not very wide. I was feeling a lot of downward pressure and the intensity was building, but nothing was unmanageable yet. I decided to try the tub though, just in case it helped take the edge off, but it didn't. I couldn't get comfortable, and the heat didn't do much for me. While I was in the tub though, Karl started playing music for me. A month or two ago, we discovered a song that we both really like. It's called The Last Goodbye.

I had listened to it over and over in the last few weeks of pregnancy and found it comforting. As I contracted uncomfortably in the tub, I noticed for the first time the deep soothing bass notes. They're really subtle and when you just listen to the song you don't really notice them. Something about being in another room, or just being in tune with a different frequency really enhanced these particular notes for me. I felt like it was her frequency, that she has a deep, even dark quality to her. It centered me, grounded me and helped me to refocus. I listened to it a few more times, not the whole time, but the feeling stayed with me.

I found I was actually more comfortable sitting on the toilet than I'd ever been before. In all past labors, the toilet always made me hurt more, but this time it was kind of nice. I had the bidet to my left and a ¾ wall on my right, so I had plenty of support I could prop myself up with during contractions. My body was also pretty busy with trying to get rid of anything in it that wasn't necessary, which made sitting on the toilet a wise choice as well as comfortable one.

Still feeling a bit restless, I paced back and forth from bathroom to bedroom. Toilet to side of the bed. I found kneeling beside the bed, or on the bed to be most comfortable. I was humming at this point through contractions, and Karl would come to my side and apply counter pressure to my back, or give me a nice double hip squeeze. He was keeping good music going on youtube. At one point I picked up my phone to check Facebook or something and realized it was the last thing I wanted to do, so I shut the phone off completely and tossed it across the bed. I hadn't really been keeping an eye on the time, but I completely lost track of time at that point.

It couldn't have been much more than an hour or so after Karl got home that I started to really struggle through the contractions. My humming was turning to throaty vocalizations, and I was starting to feel a little panicky at the peaks. Again, just afraid of it getting worse, and afraid of the pain, not of the process. As I knelt over the little steps in our bathroom that go up to the window, next to the tub, I suddenly realized that I hadn't really prayed about my pain or my fear, and one of the things I had desired most about this intimate birth experience, was to have it be a spiritual experience.

So, in that moment, I began to pray. I prayed that I would be attended to by any who was available to help. That here in the land of my foremothers, I would be looked after by those who came before me. That through even the atonement of Christ, the pain I was feeling could be lessened, and that the feelings I was having could be put into perspective for me. That I would feel the purpose, that I would feel the work, and the pressure, but that I wouldn't feel it as pain. I asked for peace and comfort, and I received it.

I became quiet. I become focused. My mind was at rest, and I even began to smile a little during contractions. I found my way back into the bedroom, and counterpressure stopped being beneficial. Instead I would reach for Karl's hand, and it would be there, ready for me to squeeze. I have always labored noisily before at this point, yet this time I was able to find comfort in my own silence.

I contracted several times in the bedroom, then would make my way back to the bathroom. Soon I began to bleed, which is my indication that transition was beginning. I typically begin to bleed at around seven centimeters or so, so I knew we were getting to the end. I was still having a pretty easy time coping. A contraction would come, and I would pray to "feel the pressure, not the pain," and for "help to be by my side."

I made one more trip to the bathroom and brushed my teeth. I don't really know why, I just felt like I should. After that I didn't leave the bedroom again. I also lost all my clothes, except my small stretchy bra. We'd already let the kids have tablets upstairs and asked that they not come down anymore.

Daniel had come down during one of my earlier vocal contractions and with a very concerned look on his face asked, "What is going on in here?" I smiled at him and told him I was fine, and that I was going to be having the baby later. He smiled real big and got excited. I had watched numerous birth stories and videos on youtube with him. He is fascinated with the human body, and all of it's functions, and I wanted him to not be afraid of the noises he might hear coming from me.

Apparently, that worked. But it was around then that we had them all stay upstairs. I had considered having them involved and witness the birth, but alas, I am who I am, and didn't want any of them near. I needed silence. I didn't need questions, and I didn't want to be concerned for them and their emotional states. Miraculously, they listened and nobody disturbed us.

The bed was already lined with plastic and we had lots of chux pads. We spread the chux pads on the floor and on the bed. My knees were getting sore, and the intensity was rising. The downward pressure was beginning to become unbearable and I began to have a deep burning in my lower back during contractions. That was probably the hardest or most painful part, the burning in my back.

I began to feel a little irrational. I didn't know what to do. I didn't know where to go. It's funny, because my sister Holly said the same things out loud when she went into transition with her last baby. It's not an uncommon thing to say, but it's always a funny thing to hear when you're helping a woman give birth. Where else would they go? What else should they do? But here I was, asking the same questions. "Where do I go? What should I do?" I think the deeper meaning of my questions were, "How do I make this end?" and "What position is going to feel the best?" But in the primal state it is hard to be more specific.

Being upright was eventually too intense for me. Logically, I know, and even then I knew that it was a great position to push from. Gravity can help immensely, but I've never had a difficult pushing phase. Even with Violet who was face-up didn't take more than 15 minutes to get out after I'd found a good position to push from. So, throwing logic to the wind, and all the pillows on my bed to the head board, I pulled myself up onto the bed and propped myself up into the semi-reclined position one typically assumes in a hospital bed.

Karl recognized where I was and what was going to happen and got a chux pad up under me and then several more all around me. I had two or three contractions with him bracing my feet so that I had something to strain against. I wasn't pushing, but my body was beginning to. I remember him trying to get into an optimal position, and he wasn't moving much, but it was too much for me. I told him to stop moving. He did. And then with great force, my water burst.

It took me by surprise, and while having my water break has always felt really, really good and relieving in labor's past, this time, while I did notice a slight feeling of relief, I also knew that it meant the baby was now coming. I did remember to ask if it was clear, and he answered that it was "clear as a bell." I laid there with my eyes closed, breathing and relaxing as much as possible before the next contraction. I let the next one come, rise and fall and stopped myself from pushing, but with the second contraction after the flood, my body began to do the work for me.

Silent no more, I grunted and roared. I only pushed when my body pushed. There were no long held counts of ten, just very determined and efficient bursts of downward motion. I could feel everything. I felt her pass my cervix and enter the canal. Karl told me when he could see her head. I felt her crown and felt the burning, and I remember to not push when it burned badly.

I exclaimed loudly, "I HATE THIS!" I remember thinking that I wasn't quite ready to be doing this part yet. I reached down and applied counter pressure to myself to help me not to tear. I asked him to do the same, but that was one thing I had neglected to teach him about. He didn't know where to put his hands, first putting them on my hips, then on my belly. When I was able I told him, "no, here!" And he did, and it helped. I was leaning to the left, holding on to the post of my headboard, and reaching for the bedside table with my right hand. It was only one contraction, but it felt like an eternity was passing. She crowned and then her head was born.

I remember pleading, "Help me!" In my head. I wanted him to pull her out for me, but then I remembered that you're not supposed to do that! I remembered that I still needed to push, that I had to do it on my own and that she was waiting for me, so I waited for the next downward motion and pushed with it. I felt her turn and slide. Karl was there the whole time, supporting her head, catching her slippery body and rolling her over to untangle the long cord that was wrapped around her body.

She let out a substantial wail and cried with vigor. I audibly sighed with relief and smiled. I had done it. It was finished. I felt so much better! Just a lingering burn, but I was still alive, and my body was in one piece, contrary to the way I had felt just moments before. I asked for just a moment, to get my bearings. Karl held her safely in his hands, and looked her over quickly, and found her perfect, then placed her on my chest when I was ready. He checked the time and it was 6:47 p.m. She was warm, and wet. She had no vernix and no blood on her body. She smelled fresh and organic, and felt strong and robust.

She cried while I rubbed her back and talked to her. Eventually she settled down. Karl kept an eye on me, and my bleeding and began to change out the wet pads. He brought me a warm cup of tea with herbs that help the process of getting the placenta out and can even help staunch bleeding. I drank it down easily. I felt great. He boiled string and sterilized the scissors we would use to cut the cord and I basked in the heavenly feeling of oxytocin and warm new baby on my chest. When she felt like it, she began to bob her head to find her new source of sustenance. I helped her find what she was looking for and she latched on, perfectly the first time and nursed successfully.

After about 45 minutes we cut the cord. I was feeling impatient about wanting the placenta out. I gave the baby to Karl to hold, and I squatted by the bed to see if a little gravity would help. Then I moved to my chair to just rock a bit, and took the baby back to see if she'd nurse. Karl watched a video to refresh his memory on this stage of labor and then attended to me. He said a little prayer in his head, and as gently pulled on the cord to test it, he felt impressed to pull it slightly upward. In that moment we felt movement and I pushed slightly to help ease it out. Out it came, perfect, healthy and whole. And now I was truly done. I sat a while longer then stood and cleaned myself up and got back into my clean, dry and prepared bed.

The kids came down after that to meet her briefly and everyone fell in love. She looked like my newborn pictures, just much bigger and already chubby. I have never had a newborn that was chubby. That first night she was convinced that her life depended on being attached to my breast, which was expected. She also was still snorting quite a bit, so I didn't mind because I wanted to keep an eye on her and make sure she didn't start to struggle to breathe. In the early morning hours I tried using a bulb syringe on her nose to just see if anything would come out. It seemed to help a little, but she thought I was trying to murder her. At around four in the morning, she figured out that she could in fact sleep while not attached and we both got some good rest.

In the past it was frustrating that Karl could so easily sleep through these first nights and even the piercing cries, but it no longer bothers me. The night is just ours. We are dependent on each other only. All my fears of pain, and breastfeeding, and exhaustion have gone, and it's just me and my girl now every night. My little Juniper Jane Clinger.

Three Days in Labor
Submitted by Kala McGillicuddy

LAKEWOOD, WA USA
July 2018

I had been trying to conceive for seven months and miscarried right before I conceived my son, so I was tracking my temps for ovulation and calculated my due date based on that. I was due July 15th and he was born on July 15th! I did have prenatal care during my pregnancy. I moved to a different city two weeks before my son was born, so I was no longer in their area for care. This was my 6th pregnancy and 5th live birth, he is my rainbow baby!

On July 12th I started having regular contractions (these were different from the prodromal labor I had been having for three weeks). They were getting stronger and closer together. My friend was over and she helped me fill my birthing tub. After the tub was filled my contractions started to simmer out.

I was able to get some rest between contractions that night and then woke the morning of the 13th with strong consistent contractions. I had my mom and mother-in-law come over, and my water broke at 6 p.m. I continued to have contractions and my pubic bone was hurting severely with each contraction, which told me his head was pushing on it (posterior position). I tried laying down and contractions died down enough for me to rest again, and I woke in the early morning with strong consistent contractions again.

I went for a walk and was extremely emotional, which meant transition. I headed back home to sit on my ball thinking it would help with my pubic bone pains. At this point my contractions started to feel "pushy" but I knew he was still too high and stuck on the front of my bone. I tried leaning back during contractions, but it was not helping. I felt at that time that I had done every position I could think of, except for laying on my back.

So, out of desperation to move him off my bone to get into my pelvis, I laid on my back on my bed. As soon as that happened I had a really strong contraction and could feel him slip past my pubic bone! After that, my body pushed and it started hurting my back. I had my husband put the birthing ball on the bed so I could lean on it while on my knees. My son was born just a few pushes later, and my husband handed him to me. His head was coned to the side and he had a bruise on his forehead, which indicates that he was crooked and pushing against my bone. He was born at 1:23 p.m., three days after my contractions started!

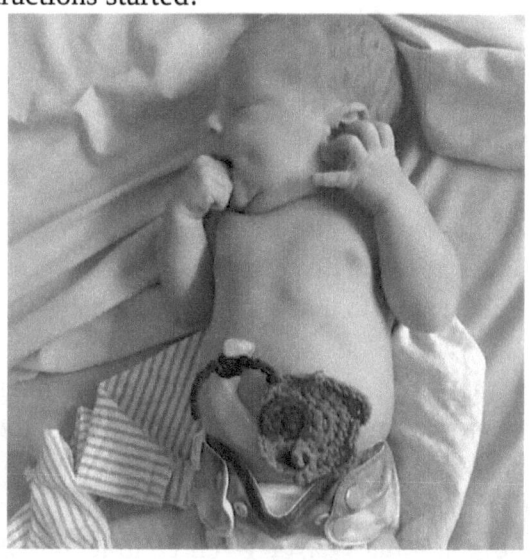

The Power I Always Had: My Home Birth Journey
Submitted by Angelica Stevenson

SO MOST OF YOU know I was pregnant and had a baby, a beautiful young lady. What most of you don't know is that I had her at home with the help of my awesome husband, Allen Stevenson.

The reason why I wanted to do a home delivery is because I kept learning, studying, and researching for myself the dangers, and unnatural ways of the hospital and it's staff. My last son was delivered in the hospital, however, he came out before they had time to hook me up to anything. The midwife lied to me about his umbilical cord, and when I saw him being circumcised that was it. I wanted all natural for my next baby.

Hubby was reluctant. He was worried of course, had questions, etc. So, I made sure to watch at home birth videos of different types of deliveries including breech. I joined this awesome Facebook group where women have babies at home and they help, assist, and encourage each other. Some women in this group were nurses, midwives, already had one or more home births. There was a woman who had 6 or 7 home births and she was pregnant again, and was experienced as well. I read up on lotus birth. I downloaded a guide for myself and for those who would be there to help me. And I bought a lotus birth kit.

I was scared at first to be honest, and other people's fear didn't help cause I took it on. However, as I began to study more, learn more, and connect more with the women of the group I began to feel more empowered, encouraged, inspired, and motivated. Women have been having babies for years way before hospitals. And their fears were no longer my own.

I went into labor in the middle of the night of July 23. Hubby and I did the deed, so I woke up with contractions and needing to poop. I thought nothing of it, it's happened before. However, when I was on that toilet and the contractions weren't stopping, getting stronger, more painful and a minute apart, I was like, "I'm about to have this baby." I had to yell at Allen a few times before he got out of bed.

I got off the toilet, walked around, thinking should I call people now, is this labor, gotta go potty again, etc. etc. I was telling hubby to get the strainer for the placenta because we were having a lotus birth. I told him to get the papers from out the car about lotus birth, the guides on what to do. I sent the texts to people. Had to go potty again and this time I was like, "Shoot, the baby is coming." I had a dream a few weeks back that I was on the toilet going potty and the baby's head came out. I was like nope not happening so even though I had to poop, I refused to have the baby on the toilet.

So, I grabbed our extra shower curtain, went in the living room, laid it out, got on my hands and knees and started pushing. I had to yell at Allen to get off the phone cause she was coming. I pushed once and she was half way out. Allen was like, "Push again." I told him, "Don't rush me."

Second push and she was out. All in all, the total amount of time between me waking up and having her was probably like 45 minutes. (And thankfully no complications or any of the worries/concerns that Allen had.) There was less blood than at the hospital, and a woman mentioned because I wasn't stress bleeding like I was at the hospital. Because it is stressful in the hospital. And at home it was more peaceful with just me and the hubby. I was sad cause our other three little people weren't awake and they've been waiting and watching videos with me. So when they did wake up and she was there they were like, "Is this baby? Baby came out of your yoni." It took a few days for them to get used to her.

She was born on a Saturday and the umbilical cord came off on Wednesday. It was hard and the cord was starting to lift up, and come off by itself from her belly button, so I knew it was getting ready to. However, with her cord it snapped of while we were sleeping and she cried. It hurt me so much and confirmed even more that when they cut the baby's cord when they are first born it hurts the baby, the baby feels the pain. There are different things you can do with the placenta. I chose to dedicate it back to the earth.

The afterbirth was painful, not going to lie. With each child it gets worse. You know how the staff pushes on your stomach? That's not needed. When I fed my daughter, my uterus contracted on its own and that assists in the process. Yes, it may be slower, however it's still natural and I'll take natural any day. No, it's not required to put her in a incubator. My own body heat warmed her along with towels and blankets. Shout out to my sister, Schmeeka Grayer, for bringing us more towels cause we didn't do laundry yet. And hey, if she didn't or wouldn't have made it, I would have used shirts. Whatever works, you know?

All in all, she is my healthiest and most natural baby and delivery. And it was so cool to watch the natural process of her opening her eyes and getting used to her surroundings without them putting that stuff on her eyes.

For all those who may start popping off at the mouth thinking you know something without studying and doing the research for yourself. In Nebraska it is not illegal to do a home delivery. And it is not as hard or horrible that people make it out to be. Know yourself, you have the strength, power, and courage within to do this. Study and research for yourself, so that your baby can be the healthiest and best from jump. We as women have been giving life since the beginning of time, and it's time we take it back. I've even learned some more new information that I look forward to teaching, sharing, and passing it on, to make delivery even easier and wonderful for women.

I am very thankful to Allen for trusting me and supporting me in my decision to have a home delivery. And also for cleaning the poop off my foot. I love this man, and I'm thankful he loves me just as much and more to do these things.

The Manifestation of Light & Darkness
Submitted by Angelica Stevenson

SO ON SUNDAY, FEBRUARY 11, 2018 at 7:05 p.m., our A-Team empire welcomed our new addition. A boy. That's five little people and our second unassisted pregnancy and childbirth at home. We were expecting him at the end of the month.

This labor was so different for me because all of it, the pain, the contractions were in my back, butt, stomach, hips, basically everywhere except my yoni like I was used to. Which is why I didn't know I was in labor until way later. I realized, okay, this isn't just Braxton Hicks, these aren't going away and they're getting worse.

My little people, Alex 6, Alaina 4, Adis 3, Amhra 1 were very helpful during this process. I didn't assign them anything for this delivery, so we were all just winging it together, literally.

And they did an excellent job. They comforted me, patted me on the back, gave me hugs, asked me if I was okay, stayed with me when I was throwing up and reminded me to breathe. Like my four year old daughter, she said, "Remember mom, calm down, breathe, don't scream."

I said, "Thank you, I'll try not to."

My husband, Allen, almost didn't make it in time. I was kind of hoping he wouldn't, to get that experience of catching the baby myself. However, he walked in the door just as I started to push and could feel the baby making his way and started crowning.

The little people just watched and waited with their dad. I screamed once, and my eldest daughter said, "Mom, don't do that.

You're scaring Adis and he doesn't like it." And Adis said, "I don't like that."

Now, for those who don't know, labor and delivery is not always a pretty and beautiful process. As Allen says, "It's a lot of liquid." And I had fluids and body movements coming out all three of my holes. That was hard and painful as heck, trying to push out a baby while vomiting and pooping at the same time.

And the ring of fire was no joke with this one, it hurt and burned like crazy, and I didn't do well in listening to my body this time and going with it instead of against it. I loved the feeling of pushing and delivering my first four children. However with this one, nope. Didn't love it all. Just keeping it real. I can laugh about it now, though.

Once he was out, my eldest daughter and second son went back to watching TV like nothing happened. My eldest son was a big help, like with the rest of them. And my youngest daughter. She just kept saying "Baby! Baby! Baby!" Asking him if he was okay when he cried, kissing him. It was cute.

The other main difference with this delivery was that I ended up having retained placenta in me. It took me awhile to push out the placenta cause I was tired and I think I was rushing it, forcing it cause I wanted to be done. When it did come out it was ripped. The membrane (skin/surface) part of it.

I was worried about our son, so I took a picture of it asked the unassisted childbirth/freebirth group I'm in about it. I love that group!. They advised me I could still do a lotus birth if I wanted. Just watch out for my baby getting blue in the face, seizures, fever etc. Or I could tie the cord off. He was blue in the face coming out, and it went away as time went on. So he's fine. Looking just like his siblings. I still did the lotus birth. The umbilical cord has not fallen off yet.

However, I got sick. I had the shakes, fever, bleeding was normal though. About 1-2 days later two women from the group commented on my post saying I should also worry about retained placenta in me and to check it to see if anything is missing. Just like what they do in hospitals, they open the placenta and check it to make sure it's all intact. Allen said he's seen it done before after one of our three childbirths at the hospital. So I looked up the symptoms for it because I thought it was just after birth stuff and a little extra.

This is the part where I understand why pushing on the stomach is done AND also that it doesn't have to be done as well because the body has its own natural way of expelling the rest of the blood, clots and stuff out of you after delivery.

However, in this case since there was a good possibility of retained placenta in me, Allen put his foot down and said, "We are pushing on your stomach, if this doesn't work we're going to the hospital." And I agreed, no debating or fighting this time from me because it can be dangerous and life threatening. So that's what we did, and sure enough placenta came out of me after some pushes and breaks. And once it came out I immediately felt better. Shakes stopped. My body temp started to go down, and I no longer smelt like placenta.

The next day, the little people were back to their routines and even New Baby A was back in his routine like he had in the womb. Sleep during the day or just quiet. Up at night. My eldest son helps and enjoys holding his little brother. Also helps me too, so very grateful for that.

This week has been a great break. This pregnancy, delivery, process, has been another great experience, lesson, and time to go through.

I named my son Arayn which means "a ray of light within." It came to me while I was working one night at Planet Fitness watching a storm, thinking how dark it is and about some personal issues I was going through. It reminded me that there's always light within me and waiting.

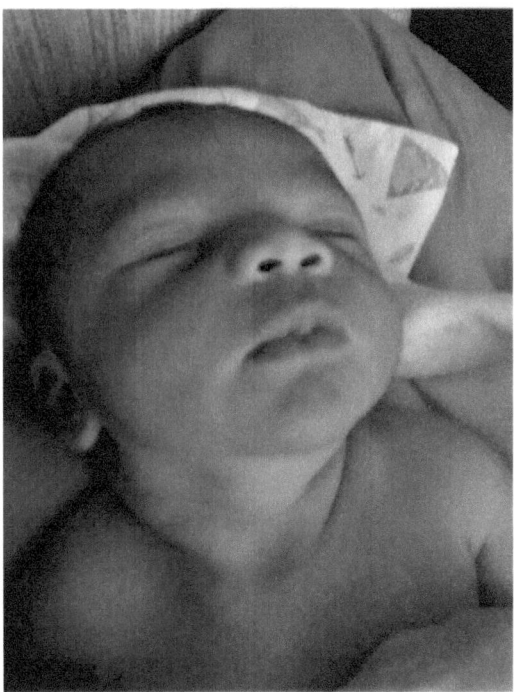

Looking at my son's face though so handsome, it was also red and bruised. I told Allen my yoni needs a break. It's beating up our babies more, and they aren't coming out with pretty faces anymore.

*Putting myself in the shoes of my daughter Amhra who was my first home birth child, and her reactions to her new baby brother, who is my second home birth baby. We resided in Omaha, Nebraska at the time of both home births.

The Freebirth of Oswin Isaac Lund
Submitted by Aerin Lund

OSWIN ISAAC
March 7th
Oklahoma, U.S.A.

After our daughter's horrific Pitocin induction, which I had been pressured into by everyone around me, I laid down the law and told my husband who had been a deciding factor in my surrendering to obstetrical care that I would not be going back to a hospital to give birth. I explored all the other options: birth center, assisted home birth, and freebirth. I chatted with multiple women about each option and decided that freebirth would be the best for me.

I had been very pregnant for several weeks by the time I went into labor with my second child, my first freebirth and first home birth. I opted not to seek any medicalization of my pregnancy, so I only saw a doctor once at 39 weeks to get proof of pregnancy for the birth certificate. After that point, I consciously resisted impatience, going about my life as normal, attending class and running errands. I knew that at any point I could have a precipitous labor and, for instance, give birth in the accessible stall in one of the bathrooms in Gardner Hall at the University of Utah where my class was. Or at the grocery store. Or at my friend's house. Or on the side of the road. I entertained many similar birth fantasies in the final weeks of my pregnancy, amused at the thought of having to tell stunned janitorial staff, professors, or university students not to call an ambulance.

Perhaps fortunately, I started having "different" (not so-called "Braxton-Hicks") contractions the afternoon of March 6th, at 41 weeks and 3 days, when I was at home. I thought I might be in early labor but put the thought out of my mind, continuing to consciously avoid impatience. I made dinner and played a favorite video game with my husband while my mom watched our two-year-old daughter. Throughout this time my contractions became more frequent, and perhaps more insistent, but never painful and certainly not unbearable. I had to stop a handful of times to breathe through them. I asked my husband if he would like to have sex to encourage contractions. We did, and during my climax I had an overwhelming surge that shattered any doubt I had about this being "it."

We played some more video games and my husband developed a migraine so we went to bed together while my mom continued playing with our daughter. I decided to go lie down on the bean bag chair because I kept shifting to get more comfortable, and I wanted to let my husband sleep so he could help me when I needed it. (Spoiler: I didn't need it.) I labored and tried to nap on the bean bag chair for an hour or so and my mom brought my daughter to me to say good night. I gave her a hug between my contractions and laid back down to continue my attempt at a nap.

After some time, I woke up and felt like I needed to go to the bathroom. I didn't want to get up, but I did. I emptied my bladder and after I wiped I decided to check my cervix. There was the bag of waters, and behind that, my baby's head. I called for my mom and said that it was happening. I felt pushy, so I pushed once and the bag of waters exploded everywhere! Then I pushed again, still hovering over the toilet, and my baby's head and body ejected immediately into my hands. My husband had heard me call for my mom and walked in just as the baby came out screaming! His cord was wrapped around his neck twice and my mom unwrapped it for me. I pulled him up to my chest and my mom said we had a boy! I couldn't believe it, so I checked, and sure enough, it was a little man child. I was overjoyed and couldn't stop hugging and loving on him, crying with happiness. We checked the time and it was 3:15 a.m., so he had been born on March 7th when I was 41 weeks and 4 days pregnant.

After a bit of time snuggling my new little baby on the bathroom floor, I felt the placenta ready to be born as well. I asked my mom to get the bowl I had set out to catch it and I squatted over it and promptly birthed the placenta onto the linoleum. I laughed and apologized to my mom for the bloody mess. We then decided to cut the cord, and I told my new baby boy what would happen and promised that it wouldn't separate us. We tied his end with the beautiful purple crocus cord tie my best friend had crocheted for him. We weighed him and he was 9 lbs 9 oz, the same as his sister's birth weight.

I then took a shower and we spent the next several days cuddling and nursing. His big sister loved to kiss and hug the new tiny baby. He never left me, as I was always wearing him in the Rebozo. We went to the grocery store when he was two days old and I returned to my class with him when he was five days old. I felt ready, energized, and healthy because his birth was so darned easy! I received multiple comments from startled friends, acquaintances, and strangers that I was "brave" to leave the house so early, and that they were amazed I felt strong enough to do so. I explained to many of them that I had given birth without interference, which is the easiest way.

On the third day after his birth, I told my husband we should probably give our new son a name, so we sat down and scrolled through baby name lists while we all snuggled and I nursed the baby. After much discussion, we decided on Oswin Isaac. Oswin is an Anglo-Saxon name meaning "divine friend," which turned out to be very fitting, especially for our little daughter. Isaac is his father's name.

I would never give birth any other way, knowing what I do now. I thank all the women who led me to this path for their hand in my decision to reclaim my female power.

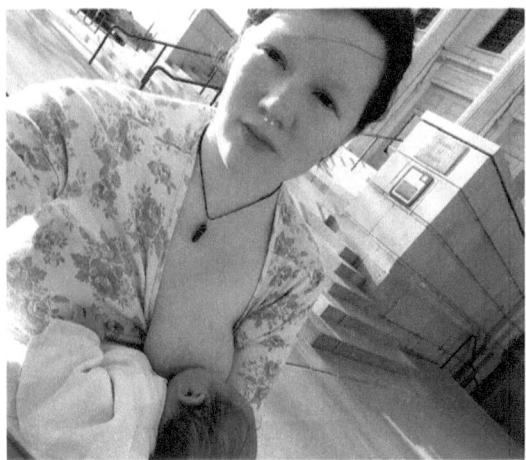

42 Weeks and Counting

Submitted by Ann W.

I WAS TWO WEEKS overdue, and other people were freaking out that the baby wasn't here yet. I wasn't worried. The previous pregnancy I was pregnant for a year and I knew that it is quite normal for babies to come at 10 months instead of 9. The only thing that was bugging me was that I wasn't having any mucus discharge. My last two I had mucus discharge throughout the third trimester, so this was strange for me.

On March 9th I had bloody show and went into prodromal labor. The contractions were getting stronger and closer throughout the day until they just stop progressing. They didn't slow or get less consistent. They just weren't going anywhere and I knew it. My husband, Jay, tried to get them to progress again by being lovable. That's when they finally stopped. We were disappointed and I felt like I let people down again (I always get prodromal labor before the birth). However, I knew that with the bloody show the baby would be here in the next few days.

The next day I was just trying to get breakfast for my kids when the contractions came so strong that I was shaking. I was texting Jay to get home now (he was working night shifts at the time and just had just gotten off of work). Soon after he had gotten home my sister came to get my kids. I was so glad she could take them. The contractions were so strong all I could do was try to rest in between, but strangely enough, they were painless.

I spent most of the day in the tub. I have no idea how I would have been able to get through the contractions without the tub. Sometime after lunch, I had to have Jay with me. I just couldn't do it alone anymore. Then I stepped out of the tub to go watch a show when my water broke. It felt like a bubble popped inside of me. I instantly wanted to get back into the tub.

That's when I started pushing. I could feel the baby descending. This baby was big. Much bigger than my other two. I remember thinking This baby is so big. I'm going to tear. I got prepared to tear when I pushed him out in one push. I was shocked I didn't tear, and he was here. At 2:25 p.m. my baby boy was finally born on March 10th, weighing 7 pounds.

Free to Birth
Submitted by Anonymous

I HAD MY DAUGHTER in early summer 2016. Her birth was an unmedicated hospital birth with a Doula, and by society's standards it went perfectly. To me, though, it brought back my rape from years before. My birth was wonderful as could be in a hospital setting, but afterwards I was hurt by my doctor as she laughed and caused more pain, intentionally with no medical benefit whatsoever. I was pushed to let my hours-old newborn cry it out, which I refused to do.

So, when I found myself pregnant with my son when she was just 18 months old, I knew I couldn't go back to a hospital again. My husband and family fought me on it, told me I couldn't do it, shouldn't do it. Anytime I contemplated giving them the power and doing what they wanted me to, I had a panic attack thinking about what could/would happen. Eventually my husband began supporting me in it. My family never did, but I didn't need them to. This birth was for me and my son, not for anyone else.

When I was 39 weeks exactly, we went to Walmart to fill a prescription. Right as we picked it up at 12:30 p.m., my water broke! We hurried to the bathroom section and grabbed a towel to protect my seat in the van with amniotic fluid halfway down my legs soaking through my pants at a very fast rate. I knew this was it, my water had broken wide open and they would NOT be resealing! When we got home, we gathered up the baby's cloth diapers and took them to my father's house to bleach them (our washer would not work for it while his would, and I didn't want the bathtub taken up with diapers if labor hit and I needed it). It seemed my body knew to wait for both the diapers to finish and for me to get home. It took us 9 hours to bleach and dry the diapers, then eat dinner and get home.

When I walked in the door at 9 p.m., I had about 15 minutes before contractions started. I was stuffing/organizing the diapers we had just gotten ready, putting away the laundry that I had put off, talking with a few friends and my mother. I kept going, having to stop for the contractions already. My husband put on the Pandora app, Celtic music played for the next 5 hours. Out of curiosity, I timed them. 3 minutes apart right out of the gate! I insisted on putting my daughter to bed myself. It was her last night as my only baby and I needed that time with her. My body slowed down, knowing that I desperately needed to hold her. I had 10 minutes with her but as soon as I slid out of her bed, another contraction hit hard.

I stayed in our shared room for maybe half an hour to make sure she was asleep but after that I was desperate for a bath. I needed the water. I got in and it instantly made things easier. Not easy by any means but easier. I had a discussion with my husband at that point about different complications, what to do if they happened, when to transfer. Soon enough I wasn't talking to anyone on the phone, I wasn't being quiet, I was roaring through my contractions! Eventually I got up to sit on the toilet for a while. I wrapped myself in towels and sat and shook through them for maybe half an hour. And then I started getting nauseous. I told my husband that transition would be soon and to get me something to puke in just in case. He came back with a shallow pot...No. Just no. So I went looking myself for something with high sides! I was not going to deal with backsplash!

Most of my labor my husband spent sleeping sitting up either on the side of the tub or on the toilet. He had pulled a groin muscle that morning and was in a good deal of pain himself so he couldn't be very supportive physically but would wake up when I started yelling to tell me it was okay, I was strong, I could do this. After transition I slept in between contractions too so it didn't bother me at all. Eventually at about 2 a.m. he tells me mid contraction he can't sit in there anymore, he HAS to go lay down because his muscle was hurting him terribly. I held up my hand because I couldn't talk, but at the end of that contraction I felt what seemed to be my fetal ejection reflex. It couldn't be, could it? There's no way it's almost over, it had just started! So I checked my cervix.

Well, I tried to anyways. I couldn't as my cervix was now nonexistent and in its place was a baby! My husband asked me what I was doing because I had told him I wouldn't be checking my cervix as my waters had broken and I didn't want to introduce any bacteria. I smiled at him and said the urge to push had started with that last contraction, he was in the birth canal and would be here soon. He made the right choice and stayed in the bathroom.

At this point I was still in the tub with no plans to get out. A couple minutes later, another contraction starts and I, looking like a giant hippo, practically flew up off the bottom of the tub onto my knees and held onto the side of the tub. This baby would not be born with me laying on my back, my body simply wouldn't have it. My body started pushing without me, and I let it do what it needed to do. I didn't try to control it, I didn't want to.

I reached down to feel my son's head be born, and while I did feel him crowning, my hand bypassed his head entirely and pressed on my perineum by instinct. With that contraction his head was born. When it was over, I sat back on my heels and rubbed his head. My husband grabbed the camera at this point and started recording it. He was asking me a million questions and I was trying to answer…But there was a head hanging out of my vagina which made it a little impossible to focus on his questions.

While I waited for the next contraction I could feel my baby turning, both inside of me and I could feel his head turning with my hand as well. The entire time I was consumed with his ear. Why? I don't know, but it felt so right to just rub his ear. Right before the next contraction I felt him kick twice, as if to say goodbye to his home inside of me forever. When the contraction started, I picked up my right leg, my body pushed him out, and I held him under the water while I guided him one handed to my other side to pick him up with both hands. He was coughing, spluttering, and sneezing so I knew crying wasn't far off. I held him at an angle to help drain out the fluid in his airways and he let out a cry within 45 seconds. What a beautiful sound!

I had a small gush of blood about 30 seconds after that, I believe it was the placenta releasing. We stayed in the tub covered with towels for about an hour waiting on the placenta, but the water got too cold for him to stay in so we moved to the bed. He had a fairly short cord and refused to be anything but skin to skin so there was no putting him down to squat and push. Two hours after his birth, we cut his cord so I could try different ways to encourage the placenta. I gave up and came back to nurse him to bring on more contractions, hoping it would help.

Finally, four hours after his birth, I went exploring. Turns out my placenta had been sitting in the birth canal what I assume to be nearly that entire time but had folded itself so it wouldn't come out easily! I got it out, and went back to cuddle my newborn and wait for my daughter to wake up an hour later. When she did, our family of four was born and I have NEVER been happier in my entire life.

Free birth gave me just that: a birth free of abuse, free of fear, free to be and have exactly what I needed in every second. I will never birth another way ever again.

'High Risk' Birth of Rainbow Baby
Submitted by Tiarra Grammer

MY FIRST PREGNANCY, I dove deep into research of informed consent. Long story short, I was pretty informed on most all the basic things of pregnancy/labor/delivery and what to expect. I knew I didn't want me or baby to have any injections, no eye goop, no coached pushing, no epidural, no circumcision, etc. Induction was something I always skimmed over because I didn't realize just how commonly it was done. I didn't think it'd apply to me any more than a cesarean section would.

However, come the end of my third trimester, my doctor began adamantly pushing for induction. His reason being was "suspected pre-eclampsia." Not even diagnosed, just suspected. The reason it was suspected? Elevated blood pressure. So I began taking and logging my BP twice a day at home for weeks. PERFECT readings. I had no headaches, swelling, or anything other than trace amounts of protein in my urine, which can easily change through the day from things like stress or strenuous exercise (like the miles and miles I began walking).

Though confident I didn't want to be induced, over the course of six back to back appointments to "check my levels," I became more and more defeated with each visit. Finally I caved. I knew it was wrong, I knew it wasn't needed, I knew I was barely 38 weeks… But this goes to show just how strong you have to be, no matter how informed, to go against your own doctor's wishes. I kick myself daily for giving into the bullying. I was not informed of any of the risks associated with Pitocin. Never.

Long story short, my delivery went "well" in the fact that I labored for 12 hours, didn't use any pain management, and delivered vaginally to a healthy baby boy. But the more I thought back on it and the more I researched artificial induction, the more and more fired up I got.

I was researching home birth the day I got home from my first birth. I knew I'd never birth in a hospital again if I could keep from it. I eventually began to consider and fall in love with the freebirth world. Freebirthing isn't about hating and refusing all medical care. It's about knowing pregnancy and birth are one of the most beautiful processes you could ever be blessed to experience. It is such a primal and instinctive process that is so delicately and perfectly designed for a woman's body. We are literally created to do this.

And to think pregnancy is a medical condition that requires near constant monitoring, permission, and intervention? That has become one of the very most ignorant and absurd statements I can imagine! We are not made to fail. This is by design. Again, we are MADE, created, formed to grow and birth a baby without the need for medical assistance! Freebirth isn't just about birthing without a "medical professional" though. It is about following intuition, first and foremost.

There are times when something is not in alignment or there is a glitch or disorder that may make unassisted or even vaginal delivery simply not possible. And we are forever grateful for the medical care we have access to in case of these emergencies, which are exactly that, an emergency. The hospital is no place for a healthy person to be simply for the fact that they are pregnant. Pregnancy should be treated as a biologically normal event that sometimes needs medical assistance. Not a medically-assisted event that sometimes happens the way it biologically should. Because MORE often than not, if you are birthing in a hospital, you are already messing with the primal and physiological process of birth. Yes, simply from being in a hospital.

Anyways, during my third trimester I went to the health department to get proof of pregnancy and to have my iron checked because I've dealt with pretty low iron my entire life. My iron was 0.2 below "recommended" levels (which - surprise! - take a few moments to research about iron levels during pregnancy and you'll be shocked at what levels really should range). So boom, there's one tick. By the end of my visit, they have labeled me a "high risk pregnancy" because I hadn't received any ultrasounds, low iron levels, previous miscarriage, length of time between pregnancies, "pre-term delivery" (Um, hello, I was INDUCED), and a diagnosis of pre-eclampsia, which I did not have.

So with those random, out of context tidbits, I was immediately labeled high risk and was told I needed to "seek immediate care."

So this is my story of my unassisted pregnancy/birth. You are capable of learning your body, determining what tests and tracking are of importance to you and your baby, and of trusting your body. I personally didn't check much unless I felt like I needed. I checked my blood pressure, used urinalysis strips, played with a stethoscope to hear baby's heartbeat and the placenta (though only ever heard baby 2 times due to position), weighed myself every now and then, monitored my swelling, checked my fundal height a couple times, etc.

You. Are. Capable. And you don't need someone of "authority" breathing over your shoulder about your birth choices. No, freebirth is NOT for everybody. Not even close. As instinctual and inevitable of a process pregnancy and delivery is, you still need to equip yourself with the knowledge and wisdom to know if/when there is a time to seek third party assistance. You must be willing to inform yourself and research any and all aspects that you can.

On 1/16, I woke up with a strong feeling tugging at my heart whispering, "are you prepared?" Being a few days past "guess date," OF COURSE I was prepared! Right?

Well, I started to take that little nagging sound more seriously when I started losing bits of my bloody show each time I used the bathroom and my waters having leaked that morning. The day went slow and contractions never really showed face despite continually losing my final plug. It was actually a bit relieving, because this baby gymnast had turned posterior and was flipping from transverse to breech all through the day! I decided "maybe tomorrow" and decided to clean the house then tuck into bed just before midnight.

I was woken up at 2 a.m. nearly on the dot to crampy contractions minutes apart. I tried to use my Hypnobabies tracks to help me sleep through them, but for some reason the Hypnobabies was NOT touching it. After an hour of trying, I decided the tracks were more of a hassle than help. I needed to be up and around, but was stuck under a dream-nursing Evan. I shot a wishful-thinking message to my mom that contractions had started and they were pretty loud and proud, but honestly thought they'd die down and just continue the next morning. I decided to track my pressure waves for fun, thinking they were irregular but they were consistently a minute long and less than two minutes apart for the 45 minutes I tracked them. General rule of thumb for hospital birth is "get to the hospital when they are a minute long, four minutes apart, for one consecutive hour." That was my kind of "OMG" moment of "This is it!"

I finally snuck away from my tot minutes before 3 a.m. and bounced on my birthing ball for maybe five minutes when I decided I'd take my ball into the bedroom in case Evan woke up. Well, the moment I stood up and took a step, water broke! I went quickly and carefully to the bathroom to check it for meconium or vernix, not only as precautionary, but mostly because COOL! It did have bits of vernix in it, and was clear waters.

At this point, I'm back in bed because Evan woke up as I was inspecting my waters. Pressure waves were still the same consistency and intensity – not needing to breathe through them, but definitely were on the verge of breath-taking! About 35 minutes in to laying Evan back down, I experience a noticeably stronger pressure wave, then pressssssuuurrrreee, POP! My waters released completely for an entire minute and a half. At 3:11 a.m., I told my mom no when she asked if I thought she needed to come yet (for pictures and support). By 3:39 a.m., I told her to come and was fairly certain baby was coming quick and furious. A few minutes later, I was sure that she was going to miss the birth! I could feel baby descending very quickly.

Just after telling her to come, I manage to sneak away from Evan (again) and run the bath. Right when I started the water, my brain got in the zone. THIS IS IT. THIS is what I've been praying for. I'm finally doing it. I had a very tiny, half-second thought of "can or should I do this?" but my confidence and faith swiped that thought away quicker than it came! I began my birthing time playlist while waiting for my mom and sisters (Evan-occupiers, curious birth-lovers, towel fetchers, photographers) to show up.

I took note that I wasn't having ANY back discomfort, so, without checking, I was trusting that baby did indeed turn and engage optimally.

I woke up Bub and Daddy minutes before 4 a.m. and told him "baby's coming, I need you to watch Evan until my sisters get here." I found it a bit humorous because as we laid down for bed, he asked if I thought he should call work to let them know he likely wasn't going to be there, but I said no. Joke's on me!

Mom and sisters arrived right at 4 a.m. as I was climbing into the tub. The intensity of my waves had graduated to "close your eyes and breathe through it" waves, still a minute long and a couple minutes apart. I had two affirmations that were the most help: "I can do anything for one minute," was the biggest help followed by "breathe sweet oxygen for baby," because I tend to hold my breath without thinking. The waves hadn't been and still weren't painful at all at this point, just an uncomfortable prolonged cramp. A hunt began to find something for me to lean back on/against in the tub, and after creative thinking, my mom brought in the Christmas gift she had bought for Evan – a rubber bouncy horse! We laughed, but it was probably the make-or-break for me birthing in the tub! Best dual-use toy ever.

I don't think I looked at a clock once from the point they showed up. I was in the zone and ready to do this. I was riding each wave like a pro, focusing completely on working with baby and my body. Each time I closed my eyes during a wave, I connected with baby on a deeper level than I'll ever begin to be able to describe. We were the only two in the room when I closed my eyes. I could see and feel every single movement, turn, and descent that baby made. It was in slow-motion and helped me immensely to be able to know how well and quickly we were making progress together. We're doing this, baby. We're working together, bringing you down slowly into this peaceful atmosphere I've created for you. This is the perfect birth that you need and that mama needs, and you are doing great. We've got this, sweet baby!

Because I wasn't watching the clock, this is a pretty wild guess but FER (fetal ejection reflex) kicked in around 4:30 a.m. I hadn't experienced FER before, but the second I felt it, it's like we had practiced for ages. I focused on giving baby oxygen so we could work efficiently together with my body. The first few waves with FER were less "productive" and more "hey, are you ready?", but by the end of each one, there was obvious and beautiful progress made!

Once I noticed FER showing its face, I reached in to see where my sweet miracle baby was – and quickly found them about two knuckles in! I ended up keeping my hand there the rest of the birth. It was probably the single most motivating and reassuring aspect of the entire process, being able to literally feel each progression with my very fingertips.

The moment I reached in and touched baby's head, I turned to my mom and said "this baby is a boy!" which, if you know me, was utterly shocking because I've been swearing up and down that this baby is a girl! It was such a surreal moment…I knew not by physical touch, but by the emotional connection I made with baby, finally getting to feel their sweet newborn head for the first time ever, not even born yet!

At this point, it didn't take long for baby to come down quickly. My waves up to this point hadn't increased in intensity any more than a good, strong cramp aside from being coupled with the FER pressure. They were coming a bit closer together, maybe a minute apart at this point.

One wave pushed baby down just to the opening then back, then the next quick wave crowned baby in about three FER pushes. I felt zero ring of fire, and even talked straight through the crowning to tell my mom "baby is crowning." I felt around baby's birthed head just to ensure baby was, in fact, anterior – yes! Incredible how our bodies work with our babies without need for external intervention or permission. My mom hollered for Levi to come in once baby was crowned, he came quickly! I asked if he wanted to touch the head and he said no, haha!

My body was giving me a break to give baby oxygen and to stroke the sweet little one's head. This resting moment before the big hurrah was only minutes long, but long enough for me to gather my thoughts and realize I am DOING THIS!

Finally, at 5:00 a.m. on the dot, I inwardly felt baby begin to turn and a wave begin with one last beautifully effective FER, and baby slips out quickly into the water. I began to bring baby up and unlooped the half-looped cord from their neck, and placed baby on my chest. We did it! I rubbed baby's back and was on cloud nine. After a moment of rubbing, I instinctively pulled baby up and suctioned baby's nose with my mouth and spit it into the water, then flipped baby back down and continued rubbing. My brain was going to ask someone for the Nosefrida to suction, but I guess my body had a different idea! It happened so quickly and instinctively.

I tried nursing baby, but baby wasn't ready to latch. We finally took a moment to check the gender and, as I said not long ago, it's a boy! Daddy was very excited, and I was just in my birth high, so emotional. Tears came and I just sat in the tub of blood, vernix, and meconium, smelling baby's head telling him we really, really did it. This is the birth I so desperately needed. It went absolutely perfect. THIS is what I needed to heal. I remember looking up at the now-relieved Daddy and told him with tears running down my face "I told you I could do it!"

At first I suspected that I ripped the placenta from my uterine wall when I pulled bub up because his cord was shorter than I anticipated, but after inspecting my placenta, it is indeed whole and perfect!

The placenta delivered within ten minutes, and by nearly 6:00 a.m. I was ready to cut the cord and go rest on the couch. We tied it off and Daddy cut it. Once cut, Evan came in to meet his new brother. Tired man was a bit confused, but nonetheless I could see in his face that he knew what just happened. We made our way to the couch where baby rested and finally latched to the breast, so perfectly! Evan got to hold him and by that time, he was so happy to meet this new tiny squish! He was very gentle and was overjoyed to have someone to look at and play with while nursing.

Our sweet rainbow baby, Reid Nolan, was born into my hands in the most peaceful atmosphere I had to offer at 5:00 a.m. January 17,

2019. He was born in exactly 3 hours from start to finish, each and every minute making such perfect progress to allow me – and him – the healing birth I so desperately sought. And I did it. We did it.

And to those who harbored the negative stares, whispers, and gossip... look at me now. I did it.

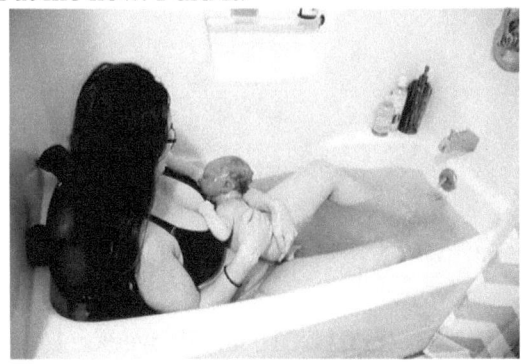

photo credit: Misty Moffitt @Moments by Misty

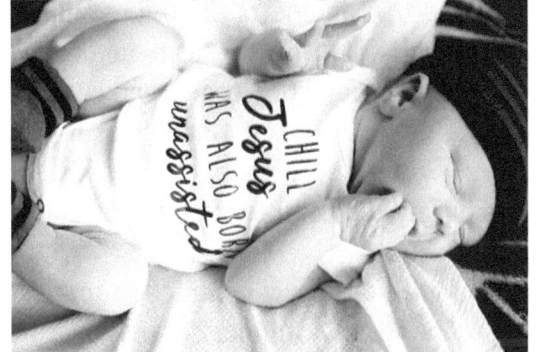

photo credit: Misty Moffitt @Moments by Misty

Family Birth is the Best Birth
Submitted by Anonymous

I WENT TO BED on 03/01/2018 at 40 weeks 1 day gestation at around 11 p.m. I woke up at 1:30 a.m. having a strong contraction. I went back to bed and had another at 2:00 a.m. and every half hour after that almost exactly. I tried to sleep in between a little bit, waiting for them to see if they got closer together. I had bloody show at around 4:30 a.m. At 5:30 a.m. I finally got my husband awake telling him it must be real because of the bloody show. He began swaying with me during the contractions. I turned some music on to sway to.

I used the bathroom after every contraction to clean out. At 7:15 a.m. they started coming at 2 minutes apart but a little bit shorter (about 45 seconds). I did some squatting before I went to the bed to kneel for awhile. I really used my birth affirmations reminding me to breathe through the contractions. Hubby was applying counter pressure each time. I ended up moving to the empty pool around 8:30 a.m. (no water, just for ease of cleanup). Contractions started getting harder and I felt to see if I could feel baby and I had a cervical lip and bulging waters.

After a few more contractions I felt again and ended up popping the waters by accident. Contractions got even more intense after that, and I was about to slowly push the cervical lip out of the way during each contraction. I tried not to push baby out as much as possible, but I could feel FER (fetal ejection reflex) kick in because it felt like I was vomiting a baby downward.

My husband kept telling me how amazing I was doing, and he was doing great keeping me breathing. At 9:20 a.m. baby's head was finally born. It took another four or five contractions to get the rest of him out at 9:33 a.m. I sucked the yuck out of his nose and mouth, and he started crying after a few minutes. My 6-year-old daughter, 5-year-old daughter, and 2.5-year-old son happened to hear my moaning and had come into the room and they got to see baby come. Although they did comment a lot about how stinky it was. Placenta was born at 9:50 a.m.

My husband was the most amazing birth partner ever! He really stepped up and went with me through this every step of the way, while keeping the kids entertained enough to not be in our faces. I'm so proud of him and fell even more in love with him. Born 03/02/2018 9:33 a.m. at 9 lbs and 20 inches long. This labor was longer than all my others by 2.5 hours, and he was my biggest baby by 1.5 lbs!

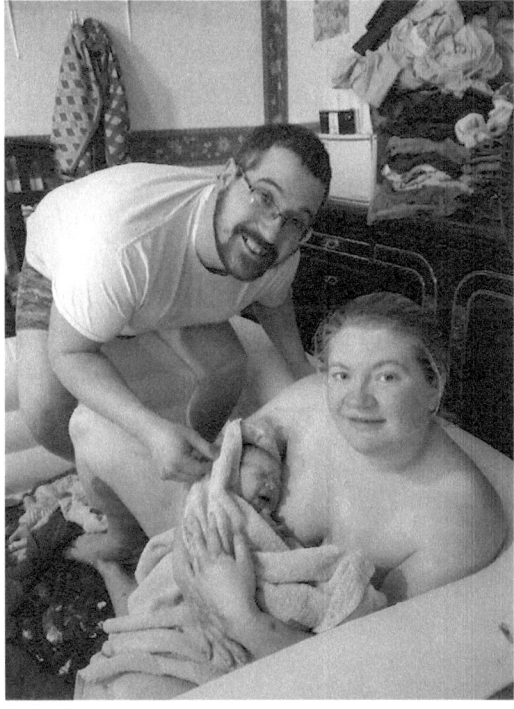

Birth Works

Submitted by Alyssa Sampson

I LIVE IN CANADA, and due to some issues with our local midwives mine quit when I was 39 weeks. I had already been considering not calling her unless I needed to transfer to a hospital, so it didn't really affect me any. I had 3 previous babies, and 4 previous miscarriages, so I felt confident.

Just after 41 weeks, after only a 2 hour labor, I birthed my 3rd daughter in our living room with my mother, my husband, and our eldest daughter (who had just turned five) present. I could feel that I was pushing intentionally, so I started breathing and relaxed my muscles and let my body take over because I could tell if I continued she'd come too fast and I'd have a bad tear.

She came out with minimal tearing, which I let heal naturally. It was the most amazing experience of my life. My family was extremely supportive, despite having never done anything so against the grain before, and my husband would tell complete strangers about our newest "adventure" and they'd just be in awe at my bravery. I don't think bravery has anything to do with it. I trusted my body, I trusted my family and I trusted my baby.

An Absolutely Perfect Freebirth
Submitted by Stephanie Martinez

I HAD A FEELING he was gonna come that day. I had even been telling everyone that the twelfth was my due date, rather than the date my midwives gave me of the sixth. So, on the eleventh, I knew I wanted to work on getting him into a little bit better of a position. Lots of walking and hip circles on the yoga ball. I had a ton of downward pressure throughout the day. I knew he was trying to work his way down, but he was sunny side up, which didn't make it easy for him to slip his head into my pelvis.

That night, we put the boys down for bed. They had a long day (with no nap for the two year old), so I knew they'd go down easily. At 10:12 p.m., I got up to go pee one last time before I tried to sleep and my water broke on the toilet! What a rush of adrenaline knowing that this was it. I was SO excited, but also knew that it could still technically be days before contractions picked up.

Deep down, I knew that it was going to progress much more quickly than that, but either way, I knew I needed to rest as much as possible before the marathon began. I rested and even fell asleep for about 20 minutes before my 2.5 year old came into bed to cuddle back to sleep with me at 12:30. I cuddled with him until he was asleep enough for me to sneak out. I went and laid on the couch as contractions intensified.

During contractions I went on all fours with my chest on a cushion propped on the arm of the couch. Between contractions, I kind of nuzzled into the corner of the couch with my legs propped open. I knew contractions were picking up and I made a goal of letting my partner, Shawn, sleep until 2 a.m. before waking him to fill the birth tub. I made it til 1:56 before calling for him.

He came out and started filling the tub that was already set up in our kitchen. Apparently, our house doesn't have hot water for very long at 2 a.m. in December. Who knew?

At this point, contractions were really starting to pick up and I knew I wanted to get in the water. I've never had a birth tub, but I knew that the water was going to bring relief. I agreed with Shawn to just get in the birth tub even though it wasn't filled up all the way. It had a hose with cold water filling it up while Shawn had four pots of water heating up on the stove that he added in slowly one at a time. The temperature felt good.

I started out on my back in the water and it just wasn't working for me. I knew I needed to be on all fours or something forward facing. I finally found my spot and didn't want to move from it. Frog-legged with my face shoved into the side of the birth tub, bearing down and biting a towel during contractions and then hanging over the edge of the pool while resting.

It was incredible being so aware of what was happening inside my body. I would bear down with contractions because it brought the most relief, but it was different from pushing. I could tell that baby was ready, but my cervix wasn't. Bearing down was working to open my cervix.

During transition, I definitely yelled out, "I can't do it!" And Shawn never hesitated in telling me that I can and I am. At one point I consciously chose to stop myself from finishing those negative sentences. It changed to thoughts and words of encouraging the baby down and telling him I couldn't wait to see his face.

Overall, the hardest part during the entire labor, the part that made me feel like I couldn't do it, wasn't the "pain" of contractions or the fear of what if's. It was when the contractions made it hard to breathe. The baby had been riding high for so long during pregnancy and he was so big, that even if/when he dropped down, the tightening of my core felt like it put so much pressure on my diaphragm and lungs.

This is where I have to give so much credit to Crossfit, Primal Reset, and Birthfit (and my previous labor experiences). Over the past year I had been learning about breathing through workouts, breathing to combat the nervous system during fight or flight, and breathing to increase intra-abdominal pressure. Without some of this knowledge, I might have feared passing out or not getting enough oxygen. But I took control and resisted panic.

Now, my favorite part- I knew I was past transition. My contractions were more focused and held more purpose. My rest between contractions was dream-like. Legitimately like imagining deer leap through forests dream-like. Next thing I knew, I could feel him coming down through the birth canal. I could feel exactly where his head was at before he was crowning.

And then, he was crowning! Hello ring of fire, my old friend! With my most recent birth, the ring of fire was so unbearable that I intentionally pushed Malachi's body out with one push. I wasn't about to have that insane burning feeling for more than one contraction. So, naturally I thought that as soon as I felt that ring of fire I could get this baby out in one push. Wrong. And not for lack of trying. I had to let go of that idea quickly and not be afraid of the pain. And once I did, it wasn't even painful. Little pushes and his head slowly descended til Shawn could see his sweet face. Finally, his whole head was out. I knelt there, hanging over the edge of the tub with his head out of me and the rest of his body inside... now what?

Shawn helped me lean back on my left knee while I put my right leg up into a side lunge position. And then switched legs. I felt slight concern that his shoulder was stuck, but Shawn and the baby were both so calm and confident. Meanwhile, the baby was KICKING me inside to work his way down and out. It felt like he was going to kick me straight up out of the water. He was so strong and it was such a crazy feeling.

We finally found a position that worked. I can't remember exactly if I was lunging or squatting, but I was leaning back while Shawn supported some of my weight and I was able to tilt my pelvis forward. One final contraction and push- from me and from baby- and he was out! Shawn calmly scooped him up out of the water and handed him to me. There he was! In my arms. On my chest at 4:21 a.m. Absolutely perfect!

After notes: His color was good, his breathing was good, I birthed the placenta and we headed to the birth center at 7:30 a.m. to get all checked out. Good to go and home by 10 a.m. with our new little family of five! 8 lb 5 oz and 21" long. Head circumference: 13 3/4" Chest: 14.5" (hence why it took a little longer to get the rest of his body out!)

The Successful Freebirth of Baby J
Submitted by Natalie Holden

NAMES HAVE BEEN CHANGED.

From the moment he was conceived I knew I was going to have my baby unassisted. It was a decision I had come to 8 months before when I was pregnant with his brother who I miscarried (baby J was conceived on that baby's due date, amazingly enough) and had been preparing for ever since. My preference would have been to have a hands off, non-interfering midwife present who can let birth happen unhindered but is available if needed, but that wasn't an option for us, so I truly felt that a freebirth was the next best thing.

I had a low involvement pregnancy, seeing a midwife regularly in the third trimester only and had just one ultrasound at 35 weeks to ensure the placenta would not be an issue, and it wasn't. I ate well, exercised moderately, educated myself on as many aspects of birth as I was not yet familiar with, and surrounded myself with positive birth messages to counter the lifetime of bombardment in our society that teaches that birth is only safe when highly medicalised (which I have never been in agreement with in the first place but the influence is still there).

My daughters were both born at 42 weeks by my own dates (though not quite that late by the ultrasounds I had with them) so I wasn't expecting to go much earlier than that with him (by the way we didn't *know* he was a boy but I was quite sure he was from the moment I knew I was pregnant). But I was still hopeful he would come a little bit before 40 weeks when a photographer friend would be able to attend the birth.

At 37/38 weeks my husband wanted to set up the birth pool for a trial run to know how long it took to fill, and know if we would have any issues with the hot water running out etc. My girls loved having their bath in it before bed, and once they were asleep I had the most luxurious soak in it as well. It was such an empowering, inspiring experience being in the pool, imagining myself laboring and birthing right there, in the peaceful stillness of the night. The following day before the pool was cleaned and dismantled I decided to hang up birth affirmation buntings made by the women at my mother blessing the previous weekend (and some by my daughters and some I made as well). I added fairy lights and re-purposed the maternity gown I made and wore for a photo shoot to complete the perfect ambiance. But knowing how unpredictable birth is I also decided to decorate our bedroom a little bit as I felt that if I didn't birth in the birth pool/dining room as planned, our bedroom was the next most likely place.

Friday March 11th, my photographer friend, Carrie, arrived in town and I met with my Doula, Sarah, one final time. She brought some massage oils with clary sage for me to use for the duration of my pregnancy and labor. That afternoon I massaged some of it into my belly and ankles and that evening I started having very mild and irregular contractions. They fizzled out about 2 a.m., but I was also losing little bits of plug along with them so I was feeling hopeful they were doing something and just maybe I would be having a baby while Carrie was in town after all.

I had a couple mild ones throughout the day but nothing to take notice of. Saturday and Sunday night. I also had mild sporadic contractions for a few hours until I went to bed. I was applying the oil with clary sage to my belly a couple times a day, and to my ankle pressure points in the evenings before bed.

Monday afternoon we were at the grocery store when my 4 year old asked if we could buy a cake. Normally, we don't do store bought sweets, but the cake she had chosen was heavily marked down due to icing on the lid and she was so nicely insisting that we needed to buy it so I agreed. We were having a picnic with my parents that evening and I said we could have the cake for dessert, but she said "no its the baby's birthday cake." I suggested freezing it until the baby's birthday, or eating it that night and then getting another cake for the baby's birthday as well but she refused and kept insisting its for the baby's birthday - tomorrow.

Monday evening I spent two hours bouncing and doing figure eights on my birth ball after applying the oil with clary sage, and overnight I was aware of some mild surges. Nothing to take notice of or affect my sleep but enough that I was aware of them when I was up to pee and I was hopeful that over the next couple days things would continue to progress. Tuesday March 15

First thing in the morning when I went to feed and water our chickens I felt something come out of me, and as my robe and legs were damp from being sprayed by the hose I couldn't tell if my water had just broken or not. When I got inside and checked I discovered a huge bit of pink tinged plug, at least 5 cm diameter. Hooray! I felt confident that within the next day or two we would have our baby for sure.

I forewarned my husband as he was leaving for work that I may be calling him home early, but that there was no point in his staying home as I didn't think things were likely to start until evening when my kids were in bed at the earliest. But about half an hour after he left for work I stood up from the kitchen table and my water broke. Not a big dramatic gush, but enough that I knew for sure it was my waters. I put on a pad and had to change it a few times as my water continued to leak throughout the day.

I didn't time my contractions as they still felt quite mild and irregular and with my first labor which had started with my water breaking I still ended up being induced 30 hours later, so I knew it could still be a while before things picked up. So, I carried on with my day as usual; made play dough with the kids, did the housework (focused more on housework than a normal day as I didn't want the distraction of a messy house when I was in active labor). I warned my girls that I had pains in my tummy that meant the baby was coming today or tomorrow (my 4 year old again said "yes, I know today is the baby's birthday.") and they would need to be a little patient with me while I was having the pains.

I thought about moving the dining room furniture out of the way and getting the pool inflated, but I felt it would be ridiculous to do it so early, and have to then keep my kids from using it as a bouncy castle.

Around 11:30 I decided to text my husband to come home at lunchtime, around 1ish, as I started thinking about how quickly my labor progressed with my second from still feeling I was in early labor with hours to go to suddenly being in active labor and having a baby within an hour, and I decided I should have him home in case that happened again. Though, immediately, I regretted having called him as I didn't want to waste his time, and I still didn't think labor was going to progress until evening.

I did also text Carrie and Sarah at some point to give them the heads up that I was in early labor and I would let them know when they were needed.

By the time he got home it was 1:30 and contractions had intensified somewhat, and I was finding myself getting snippy with the kids for bothering me during them, so I decided to send DH out with them to run a couple errands (pick up flowers and my mom's peppermint oil in case I felt nauseous). He sent a couple emails first though, and took a photo of me vacuuming cause he thought it was hilarious I was cleaning the house in labor. At 2 he was going to take the kids to the car when we decided we should probably call my Doula first so I wasn't left entirely on my own. She's 20 minutes out of town and took about 25 minutes to arrive.

When Sarah got here, I was in the middle of cooking some beef stew, and had asked my husband to attach the hose to the tap in case Sarah and I decided to inflate the pool while he was gone. I did apologize to Sarah for calling her so early cause I still didn't feel like I needed her yet. We chatted in the kitchen while I chopped veggies for the stew, and for some reason my husband still hadn't left yet with the girls. I had a couple of surges that seemed to last a really long time, followed by feeling like I had to poo. I wasn't sure if I was feeling baby move down causing the pressure, or if I really did need to use the toilet, but I decided to go try.

While on the toilet, I was hit with a really powerful surge and knew I was now in active labor. I could hear my husband and the girls on the way out the door at last, and as soon as I could speak again I called out for him not to go anywhere anymore as this was definitely the real thing now. It was about 3 p.m.

I instructed them to start inflating and filling the pool and asked for my phone to call my photographer who was on the road immediately, but got caught in after school traffic.

Meanwhile, I holed myself up in the bedroom bouncing on the birth ball with affirmations spread out on the bed. S brought me my labor tea to drink, and I asked for grapes I had previously frozen which I had to share with my 2 year old, haha. Sarah also brought me my lavender oil and smelling that during the surges really helped.

I heard Carrie arrive, but she didn't come downstairs for a little while. She came down around the time I abandoned the birth ball as I wasn't able to keep sitting through my surges, and at the same time I discarded my underwear as my pad was too soaked with leaking waters anyway. I put down a waterproof sheet and towels on the floor and stood swaying through the next few big surges. Sarah massaged oils into my lower back and applied counter pressure during the surges, and helped me focus on my deep breathing.

I had about three big surges she helped me through, and then I shouted that the pool wasn't going to be ready in time as I reached transition. Sarah ran upstairs to check on the progress of the pool, which was about half full. But I didn't have a long enough break between the surges to have been able to get in anyway.

She came back down as another surge was starting, which I had to vocalize through, and I could feel the baby descending and my body began to bear down. I'm not sure whether it was the fetal ejection reflex or whether I was actively pushing, but I know there was no way I could have *not* pushed. I said the baby was coming and Sarah lifted my skirt (yep, I gave birth pretty much fully dressed), and said she could see the head. Carrie ran to get my husband, who was still upstairs.

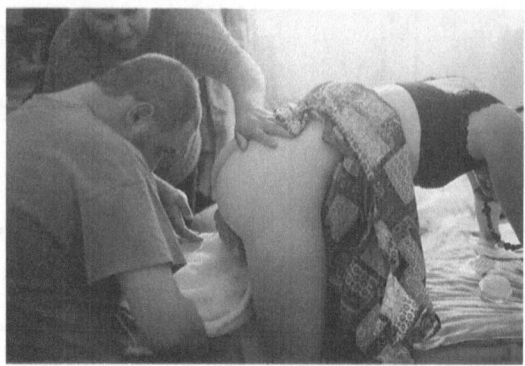

photo credit: captivatedphotogtaphy.com.au

I roared through the ring of fire, and the head was out. After the briefest of pauses my body bore down again and I roared again as the shoulders rotated and the rest of the body followed and was born into my husband's hands.

I lifted my skirt to peek through my legs to look at my baby, and I could see a scrotum! "Its a boy, we have a son!" I said over and over as I reached through to grab him and lift him to my chest. His cord was very short so it was very awkward to maneuver him through and get turned around.

He was born at about 3:45.

I just sat on the floor as it was too hard to get into the bed at that moment.

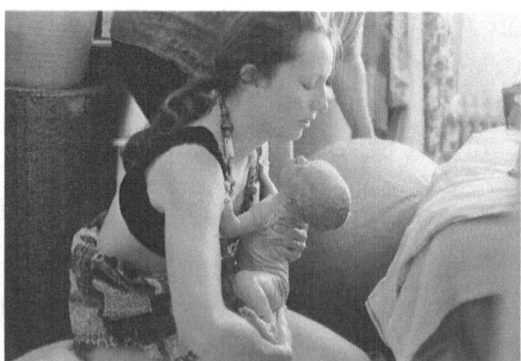

photo credit: captivatedphotogtaphy.com.au

The cord was just long enough for him to reach my breast, and Sarah and Carrie helped me get my top and birthing necklace off for skin to skin. When the girls came in to meet their brother they brought the cake with them and kept putting it directly in front of him. We offered them a piece but they said no it was for the baby, so we sang "Happy Birthday J," and then my husband took them upstairs for a piece of cake followed by a swim in the now full birth pool (no point in completely wasting the water, haha). My dad phoned around 4 p.m. to say he wouldn't be able to come over after school as he had tennis, and I answered with "You have a grandson!" which shocked him to no end, I'm sure.

I did move to the bed eventually while we waited for the placenta. My 4 year old kept coming in to check if the placenta was out yet. Eventually with much careful maneuvering because of the short cord I got up to have gravity help with the placenta, and it was finally delivered after about an hour and a half, on the tiles outside the bathroom. It was so small, but perfectly intact. My Doula caught it so it didn't snap the cord if it fell out. I only lost about 2-3 TBSP of blood with the placenta, but drank a second cup of no-bleed tea anyway.

While we were waiting for the placenta to be birthed my mom showed up to offer her assistance with the girls if necessary, so she entertained them in the living room, and seasoned my forgotten stew for us for dinner. The placenta took about an hour and a half and there was next to no blood. It was so tiny but complete. We then weighed him at 3.6kg and 54cm long, and tied the cord with a rainbow tie I had made and my husband cut the cord, which made baby J wail.

My Doula and photographer left about 6 p.m. after washing a load of towels for us, and I added some herbs to the birth pool and had a soak in it before we drained it while my husband enjoyed some skin to skin bonding.

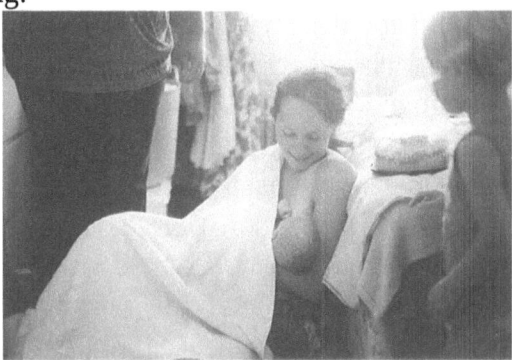

photo credit: captivatedphotogtaphy.com.au

The Powerful Birth of Kitty Rose
Submitted by Emily Cairns

UNITED KINGDOM

Trigger warning: obstetric violence

As a child, I remember thinking how unfair it was to be a female, to have the burden of carrying a child and painfully birthing that child. The concept was overwhelming. What I know now is that carrying and birthing a child is a gift. It's incredibly powerful – and it makes women powerful. I am a powerful woman.

When I became pregnant with my first child, I was living in Ballarat, Australia, and something within me led me to want a natural birth (i.e. a vaginal birth with no pain medication). After tons of research, the statistics told me that if I wanted a natural birth, then home was the best place for me. I looked into midwifery-led home births (freebirth wasn't even a concept that had registered with me yet) and, after some consideration, decided that home birth was too expensive and that I could compromise and hire a Doula, attend private birth education classes (not the hospital led classes, although I attended those too) and have enough money to spare to have my placenta encapsulated. It felt like a reasonable, logical and financially sturdy plan – unfortunately, it was the wrong decision.

What transpired on the day of Daisy's birth was traumatic, unnecessary and completely unsafe. Prior to going into labor with Daisy, I was feeling quite empowered. I had firmly navigated out of various inductions and had managed to find myself 42.2 days pregnant. However, my hospital-managed pregnancy had left me with lots of unresolved fears. The constant monitoring, ultrasounds and tests certainly had a huge influence in tilting the balance towards viewing birth with a more medical mind.

That influence was certainly noticeable when my waters leaked at 4 a.m. on May 28, 2016. They were meconium stained and it felt completely normal to get the baby monitored quickly at the hospital with a plan to head home to labor after the procedure. Once I arrived at the hospital, labor had well and truly begun and I did not feel physically able to endure another car journey back home.

I didn't feel safer at the hospital and it certainly didn't make me feel powerful – the environment felt hostile, sterile and uncomfortable. The most significant shift in mood occurred once the on-call consultant obstetrician arrived. She was more than rude, she was aggressive, pressuring me to have both an epidural and a syntocinon drip, despite having strong regular contractions and the fact that my birth plan stated not to even offer me pain relief. I refused, and asked for the bath. She persisted with the syntocinon drip and this time both my husband and I asked her to leave. I had exerted autonomy over my body and birth and she didn't like this.

By the time I was entering the second stage of birth, I had lost all autonomy over my own body – a scenario I thought was entirely impossible after 'arming' my birth team with an experienced Doula, student midwife and an informed husband. My body was touched and prodded without warning. During one (non-consented) vaginal exam, the obstetrician aggressively pulled down on my perineum and stretched it out (the purpose of this still unknown). I shouted out in pain and said 'stop' repeatedly. The student midwife placed her hand on the obstetrician's forearm and said, "Emily is asking you to stop, I think you need to stop." If you know anything about the power dynamics at play between midwives (especially students) and obstetricians, you will know that this was an incredibly brave thing for a student to say to a consultant (perhaps it will also give you an insight into how horrible that experience was in order to warrant her to say this).

Moments later, my body was cut without my consent or local anesthetic by the midwife and the obstetrician reached into my vagina and removed my baby. The aggressive way my baby was removed led to severe perineal tearing and I required 2+ hours of surgery to repair a 3B tear (2+ hours under a general anaesthetic without my baby; so much for that 'golden hour' I had so longed for). Once my baby was extracted from my body, she lay helpless at the foot of my bed. Her cord was clamped and was about to be cut before my husband noticed and shouted for her (the obstetrician) to stop. I 'awoke' from my labor haze and shouted, "Please stop. No. She's fine. She's breathing. Leave her. The paediatric doctor in the room grabbed my husband by the shoulders, looked me in the eyes and said; 'I NEED to see your baby.' I threw my hands up in the air, fell back against the bed and shouted "F*** it!" And with that, her cord was cut (by my husband – so much for the emergency) and whisked away. I felt totally powerless against the forces at play. I now know what happened to me is called Obstetric Violence.

This experience shook me to the core of my very being. The physical scars I received that day, coupled with the feelings of vulnerability lead to a PTSD diagnosis. I self-harmed, and some days it got so bad I wanted to die. However, I took my mental health seriously and with the help of various different treatments, I became well enough to move forward with my life.

I pretty much decided on a home birth for my next baby(s) before I had even left hospital after that first birth. I was now living in the UK and had access to free healthcare including the option to birth at home with NHS (National Health Service) midwives.

I had been introduced to the idea of Freebirth after hearing about my Doula's second birth (Doula for my first birth) and the seed this planted certainly began to grow.

I decided to Freebirth fairly early on in my pregnancy and the reasons I chose to Freebirth fluctuated over time. At first, it was to ensure my baby and I weren't put in a situation where we could be disrespected again (the phrase 'Fool me once, shame on you, fool me twice, shame on me' sprang to mind). However, the more I explored birth and checked in with myself, the more and more reasons to Freebirth emerged. There were certainly moments in time, particularly in early pregnancy, that made me wonder if a midwifery-led home birth would have been better (I never considered a hospital birth) but the reasons were all rooted in fear and once I explored that fear fully, it was gone.

The biggest reason for my decision to Freebirth was eventually rooted in safety. I genuinely felt I would be safest birthing this way. I totally realise that, for some, this may seem like an oxymoron but it couldn't have resonated more strongly with me. How Daisy's birth had been handled was not safe. I left the hospital with a 3B tear, a PPH and PTSD, while Daisy left the hospital with a terrible birth imprint and a strained neck which was likely from (or at least exacerbated by) the forceful way she was removed (later treated with chiropractic sessions).

Once I began to feel safe about Freebirthing, there was never a good enough reason to birth any other way. I knew I was unlikely to tear severely uninhibited at home, I knew that the uterus is far more capable than medical providers like to admit and would contract and reduce size in a safe and timely manner and I knew most babies (especially in normal, undisturbed births) would be born safely at home without the need of a resuscitation unit at hand. Normal, undisturbed birth leads to normal, healthy outcomes.

My first step towards a positive birth was having a positive pregnancy. I decided to opt-out of the free NHS care that was available and hired a private midwife. I knew what sort of prenatal care I wanted and having a private midwife was going to be the best way to achieve that care rather than navigating the NHS system. The prenatal visits took place in the comfort of my home and became a springboard to discuss fears, reservations and general birth preparation. It was a chance for my hubby and I to come together, despite busy schedules, to discuss anything on our mind about the pregnancy and birth. It was also a chance to involve Daisy with the pregnancy and normalise pregnancy and birth for her. The midwifery care I was given was the definition of respectful and woman-centred. I declined all doppler checks and only participated in the prenatal care that I wanted to have – it made for a stress-free pregnancy. I did engage with the NHS to have access to free blood tests and consented (regretfully) to one ultrasound around 12 weeks. I was lucky that the NHS care that I did receive was respectful; however, it still was very much a 'cookie cutter' type approach – one size fits all.

I wasn't the only person preparing for the upcoming birth. My husband and daughter also began their own preparations. Once a week, my husband and I would dedicate the evening to birth preparation. Over a log fire and a cup of tea, we quietly read books together, watched birth videos, learnt how to practice Hypnobirthing (breathing exercises), did perineal massage (to help soften the scar) and prepared ourselves for a beautiful birth.

Daisy was two and a half at the time of the birth and was introduced to birth throughout my pregnancy. We bought her children's home birth books and showed her positive birth videos including ones with lots of noise. I also spent time explaining that babies need to breastfeed once they are born. We revisited these two topics the most often as I felt she would need the most reassurance in these areas. Daisy was still breastfeeding throughout my pregnancy despite that fact that my milk had dried up during the 2nd trimester.

Daisy was born spontaneously at 42.2 so I didn't expect to birth before 40/41 weeks. I had regular chiropractic sessions with an amazing practitioner who had home births herself. At 41.4 weeks I decided to have an acupuncture session with the hope of restoring a good flow of Qi, giving myself the best opportunity for a swift and effective birth.

That night I started to feel a bit crampy and I thought baby would come in the next day or so. At 10p.m., I decided to go to bed. I had two surges (not cramps) in bed and - POP - something inside me literally popped and my waters broke. Not a huge gush but not a trickle either. They were clear which was a HUGE relief. My eldest daughter's waters were meconium stained and that was the first step towards the cascade of medicalisation/interventions/assaults that took place.

My hubby decided to get the birth pool/space set up and I stayed in the bedroom surging and breathing. I didn't take much notice of timings etc but I did think the surges were quite short in length. Eventually I wanted some company and went downstairs.

My mom was here, visiting from LA (I'm American) and got me a hot pack for my back and put on some birth affirmation music and aromatherapy while my husband finished the birth pool and set up the video camera (yup - caught it on tape!). My mom suggested the birth ball and I tied a birth scarf (similar to a rebozo) over a door so I could pull on it during a surge. Once on the ball, things got intense. I HAD to have hip squeezes during every surge and was pulling down on the rope like The Hulk! At this stage I began to think that the surges weren't long enough, but my mom reassured me I was exactly where I needed to be.

The pool was finished at last (the hot water turned off halfway through so it took a bit longer than anticipated) and I jumped right in. In the video you can see me in a dream-like state, eyes barely open and just totally at peace. I remember taking in my surroundings and being absolutely at peace with just my hubby and I; it felt so right. I found the water helpful but I definitely was experiencing some intense (and quite frankly painful) surges. I was gripping the side of the pool and my moans were LOUD! They varied from hollering to roaring and at times down right shrieking so loud, I woke up Daisy. My mom ran upstairs to deal with my toddler. At this stage I still didn't know I was close to birthing, so I was pleased to have someone to keep her upstairs for a bit longer and to reassure her.

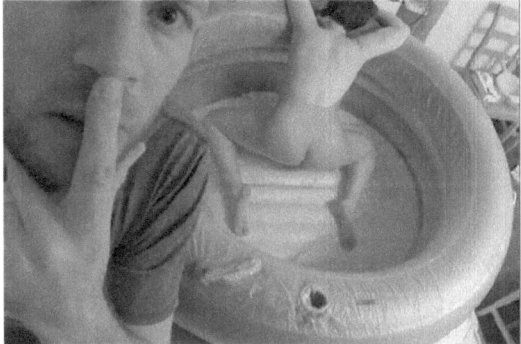

My hubby caught on tape getting the camera ready.

My hubby and I were in the pool for about 40 mins before the foetal ejection reflex kicked in. This was the most intense part of the birth experience. Everything was so primitive and natural and it felt incredibly natural to push with my body. I went with those feelings and the head crowned once and went back inside. After the next surge out popped a head – no ring of fire. I asked my husband, 'is it a head?' and he laughed with joy and confirmed it was the head.

I called out to my mom and told her to bring down my daughter and that the head was out. I then started to feel the baby rotate within me, it was an incredible feeling. I then had two 'false' surges that began but then disappeared. I wondered if I was waiting for my mom and Daisy to return? Once they both came down, the last surge began and out popped her body. My hubby tried to gently guide her up but realised she had a foot (or two) still inside and immediately stopped to allow the rest of her to be born. Once clearly out, my hubby guided her into my arms and I lifted her out of the water onto my chest. My toddler, Daisy, gave a short cry and my first words were 'look Daisy, a baby.' My baby was born at 12.25 a.m., two and a half hours after my first proper surge.

The baby looked both beautiful and healthy all at the same time! I knew immediately that she was well. I asked my mom to come and look (and with Daisy in her arms still), she brought over a face cloth and gently wiped baby's face. It was a few moments before baby made much noise, but she did give out a short cry. I later asked my mom what she thought her APGAR was and she gave her 8 at 1 minute and 10 at 5 minutes. I stayed in the pool for about 20 minutes post birth.

I had reached down around this time to feel my perineum. Because my first birth resulted in a severe tear, I was keen to assess my perineum. I felt a tear and was immediately on edge but I told myself that whatever has happened has happened and not to ruin the moment. I went back to enjoying my beautiful baby and I'm so glad I didn't ruin those precious moments worrying. It was so peacefully enjoying my beautiful baby alone, something I'm not sure I would have achieved with a midwife present. It was time to find out the sex of this amazing baby, and as a family, we uncovered the towel and found out she was a girl! My placenta had begun to separate around this time and there was some separation blood in the pool. Again, I was really pleased how prepared my husband and I had been for the birth and knew what normal versus abnormal bleeding looked like. But even more importantly, we knew not to get bogged down trying to analyse every little detail to look for signs of trouble. Being very present and in tune with our surroundings and my body was enough to keep me and baby safe. All was fine but it was time to get out of the pool.

My husband had blown up a blow-up bed in the living room next to a log fire and I tried my best to get comfortable, but the bed wasn't comfortable at all....especially with a placenta still inside me. The baby had nursed at least once in the pool so far and was having a second crack on the boob when my toddler noticed and asked for boob too! The placenta wasn't even out yet and I was like no way kiddo! I moved to higher grounds to be more comfortable and be out of the view of my piranha toddler (hehe!). I gave a couple of tugs at the cord just to see how it was going and no movement came. I tried a couple of shots of Angelica, not necessarily because I was worried about the time at this stage, but I did want to access my perineum to check for tears and get more mobile/comfortable.

After standing up to get more comfortable, I felt a heaviness in my vagina and the placenta was beginning to birth (about an hour or so post birth). I helped guide it out and after plopping it into a bowl, I then accidentally tipped the bowl over and realised the placenta never hit the ground as it was like a bungee cord from my daughter's cord. Eek!

My mom had a look at my perineum and, as suspected, I did have a tear. It started at the base of the vagina and went down in a straight line so it was uncomplicated. It did appear long but most of it wasn't deep. I did some kegels which confirmed it didn't impact my anus and we determined it was a 2nd degree. The deepest part was at the top but the rest was just skin rather than tissue, more like a graze. So although long, it wasn't deep into the muscle which was better than I had originally suspected. I had wanted to heal naturally if this occurred and after some logical thinking I decided I was going to stick with this plan.

My hubby, baby and I jumped (figuratively speaking) into bed around 4.30 a.m. and had a beautiful sleep together before our toddler woke up. We wanted a newborn check the next day and unfortunately the private midwife who was qualified to offer a newborn check was unavailable, so we decided to call the NHS to provide the check. The midwife arrived around 2p.m. the next day, and although a bit perplexed about the birth was kind and caring nevertheless.

We kept the cord attached and had planned to Lotus Birth. However, the second night our little girl wasn't settling for sleep and physically I was struggling to balance both baby and placenta while I was feeling sore. Almost exactly 24 hours after the birth, my husband and I crept downstairs and burnt her cord together. She was very peaceful during the cord burning and I felt it was the right decision. Separating the cord also meant I could encapsulate her placenta too so I felt we had the best of both worlds (a gentle separation from her placenta and placenta encapsulation for me). My milk came in that night and I woke up looking like Dolly Parton. Breastfeeding has been a breeze this time round I'm pleased to report. On the same day, we finally decided on the name for our darling girl, Kitty Rose.

I stayed in bed for about 10 days after the birth, resting, cuddling and breastfeeding my gorgeous Kitty for most of the day. The rest has been absolutely imperative to my recovery; however, on day three, I was beginning to feel nervous about how long the healing process was going to take. I began to doubt if my decision to not suture was right for me. With my mom's help, I decided to try a bit of skin glue and my mom was very heavy handed with the glue. It did feel secure at first but it also glued my bum cheeks together (that was fun pulling them apart). But on the next day, I definitely regretted the decision as the glue was extremely uncomfortable on my skin. Luckily, it began to flake off and didn't cause any adverse effects apart from a bit of uncomfortableness.

On day five, I began to feel much better down-under. It was easier to move and I was clearly making progress healing wise. My amazing private midwife who supported me prenatally came for a visit and also confirmed (and took a photo to show me) that it was definitely healing well and the decision not to suture would have also been her advice. During our prenatals we discussed natural versus sutured healing and, while sutures hold the tissue together to allow healing (and absolutely needed for complicated tears including 3/4 degree tears), they don't heal the tissue per se. And suturing does add additional trauma to the tissue.

Apart from rest, I tried to encourage healing by taking arnica, applying calendula spray to the area and using a peri bottle with an herbal mixture to wash the area after using the loo. At 10 days postpartum, I also started to apply manuka honey on top of a bit of seaweed to the area and I saw increased healing within three days of using the honey. I wish I had started this treatment earlier but the idea of a sticky honey on my perineum did not appeal at the time. For complete transparency, the very top of the tear has not fully come together but the function of my vagina (sex and pelvic floor function) has not been negatively affected and I confidently remain happy with my decision to allow the tear to heal naturally.

Overall, I can't even begin to express how amazing this experience has been for me, my family, and my daughter. Starting from conception, everything has been different to my toddler's pregnancy and birth, in an incredibly beautiful way.

My entire family has been positively affected by Kitty's beautiful birth. My husband couldn't have been prouder of me and our relationship is stronger than ever, and it has boosted his confidence as a father. My daughter, Daisy has been given a second chance to experience a positive birth that I hope will help heal the negative imprint that her birth will have left her with. Her relationship with her sister is absolutely beautiful to bear witness to. Kitty has been an incredibly peaceful and happy baby to care for and smiled within two weeks! As for me, I am the absolute epitome of a strong, confident, capable and powerful woman – the woman I had always wanted to be.

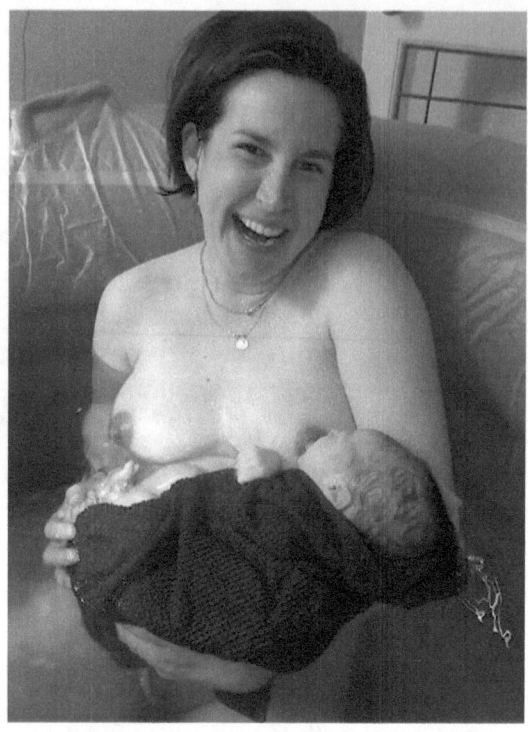

On a complete high about 15 mins after the birth. Totally in love.

Emily is a professional Doula and placenta encapsulator in the United Kingdom. You can see the services she offers and contact her at www.dsbirthsupport.com.

A Wild Island Birth
Submitted by Katelyn

KORA MIKÁ RAE BORJA

Born November 7th

First unassisted pregnancy and birth, fourth baby, conceived on the February new moon and born on the November new moon.

November 4th, Monday evening, we cleaned and organized the house as we've been doing daily since typhoon Yutu. Recovery is an ongoing process. I started feeling strong but painless tightenings all around my stomach. The sensation started to grow low into my pelvis similar to period cramps. Being that I was only 39+4 weeks (I was charting BBT aka basal body temperature), I thought I had at least another week to work on getting everything in order. I went to 41+1 with my last pregnancy. Our little Kora had different plans.

November 5th I was laying on the couch, and my waters released! There was no "pop" or gush, it was a trickle, a flowing leak. I ran to the bathroom to confirm my suspicions. Sure enough it was my water! I checked my phone. 1:27 a.m. Officially in my early birthing time! So surreal. Out of my four births this is the first time it started with my waters releasing. Such a warm feeling of excitement and anticipation knowing I'd be meeting my baby soon!

Contractions came and went, mild and totally comfortable. A gentle hug from my baby wombside. My husband had set up our birth tent out on the patio. He proceeded to inflate the birth pool and since the typhoon we've been without running water for going on two weeks now, my husband filled it with natural spring water from the shrine across the street in our village, known as the Santa

Lourdes shrine. He carried and filled by hand, twenty six '5' gallon water containers! Lugging them back and forth from the shrine to our patio and back again. There were countless obstacles standing in our way to make this water birth a reality and my husband went above and beyond. I am so deeply grateful for my man. By this time it's 3 a.m. and we are relaxing in the tent waiting for things to progress. We ended up falling asleep together and I woke up to the morning sun around 7 a.m. excited to see what the day would bring. Hopefully a baby?!

Sporadic contractions and flowing waters all day. We spent the day cleaning and waiting for any sign of baby coming soon. Turns out we would be learning a new level of patience.

November 6th. Tuesday went by without much action. More cleaning, more preparing, no sign of baby. My waters were clear with small specks of white mixed in and zero signs of infection. Feeling like I was high in a daze, moving through the motions of daily life post-typhoon. Hand wash laundry, using paper products to avoid dishes, staying cool in this tropical heat with a bucket of water to rinse off. Not how I envisioned my last days of pregnancy. Honestly, I pictured myself eating ice cream, relaxing with my kids, folding baby clothes, nesting etc. Typhoon Yutu devastated the island, our village has been without power for almost three weeks. (We have no power as I am writing this. Thanking God for generators!)

November 7th. After a restful night in the tent, I woke up around 6:30 a.m. to a tightening, but nothing painful. My two oldest, Kai and Mari, had spent the night at a hotel with their grandpa so the house was blissfully serene in the morning as Kami and Matt slept. Peace and quiet is just what I needed. The waves of tightenings were starting to roll into a consistent flow. After almost three days of leaking waters and losing small clear pieces of plug, I couldn't help but be hopeful that this was it! I started warming a few pots of water to bring the birth pool up to temp. Eventually I had to wake my husband up to pour the boiling water into the pool for me as things started to pick up from there. I found comfort and relaxation listening to the birth affirmations track for the early part of labor (from about 7 a.m. to 8:30 a.m.).

As rushes became more intense I found that I needed my focus to get through each contraction, moaning through some, staying completely silent through others. By 10:30 I was in the birth pool. This was absolute bliss! The warm water eased the contractions just enough to make it bearable. The waves started to reach around my back. Baby was descending slowly, my body looked bruised from the pressure shifting lower and lower. From 10:30 a.m. to just before noon, I transitioned hard. I kept wondering if she was really descending, wondering if my body was holding back a bit, my yoni waiting for the perfect time to melt away.

I dozed off a few times in between contractions. My face hit the water once or twice! I was surprised I could legit sleep in the midst of labor land. In a Facebook birth group a midwife whom I adore read my birth story and mentioned that I reached the sleep stage, midwives call it "resting stage" and the medical profession called it second stage narcolepsy. It seldom happens when a mother is interrupted or feeling watched.

I remember asking Matt for some more hot water, feeling the uncontrollable chills from the adrenaline running through me. Instinctively, I checked myself, and I could feel her head! It was just two inches or so inside me. Throughout the last hour of my birthing time I was falling in and out of consciousness. Occasionally checking to see if her head was still there inside me (I laugh thinking about that now). Of course it was, this baby just wanted some extra time to enter the world. A swollen cervix came to mind more than once. Ultimately, I chose to put my faith in this process, in my ability to birth my baby.

Waking up between to focus through the rush, shutting off the mind, closing my eyes, trying to soak in the calmness around me, the realness of what was unfolding. Moaning through my rushes no longer brought relief, only seemed to burn my energy. I wasn't sure if this was ever going to end! Then came the silence. A stillness. A heightened sense of awareness. A rush of adrenaline building up inside.

My daughter Kami was taking a nap, and Matt was watching me, calmly holding the space. His presence brought me peace and kept me grounded, a dose of reality in what felt like a dream. Reminding me that this is normal, natural. This is what we manifested the last ten months. Subconsciously, much longer.

Trust the process.

After getting out of the pool to use the restroom, I had Matt call our midwife friend to let her know I was in labor and assessed the details thus far. She told Matt everything sounded normal and to call back if we need anything.

I got back into the pool, and only four minutes later I started to feel the pressure to bear down. Matt asked if I wanted him to take a look since we didn't have a mirror handy, but I knew she was still tucked away inside so I told him no, not yet.

And just in that moment, Kami woke up from her nap. Matt left the tent to go to the living room to grab her (which is just 15 feet away from the patio where we had pitched the tent).

As soon as he left, I couldn't hold back anymore, I started to bear down! Oh the relief it brought. Most of the time spent in the birth pool were on my hands and knees, but as I started to push I instinctively lifted one knee and became upright in order to help guide baby in front of me once she arrived. I pushed a third time, stretching my limits mentally and physically.

Her head was finally out! The rest of her body came so gently. Such a wonderful feeling. The moment felt so long and short at the same time. She was under the water with my right hand guiding her in front of me. I had been completely silent, and yet I managed to call to Matt, "the baby is here!" He was just walking back into the tent holding Kami as I pulled our baby above the water and onto my chest.

The first push brought her past my pelvis, a second push bringing on the ring of fire, and the third and final push gave me my precious baby!

Matt looked at his phone. November 7th 12:02 p.m. We did it!

He asked if I confirmed gender. I hadn't, so we checked and sure enough, a baby girl! I felt AMAZING. Literally like magic. Waiting on the placenta snuggling with my newborn squish in the water, taking every little detail in. She nursed right away.

The final phase came simply and easily. Ten to fifteen minutes later I pushed the placenta out, and Matt put it in a bowl. I had been sleeping on my mattress in the tent for the past few days as it's much cooler outside post-typhoon. We crawled into bed and kept the placenta attached for an hour or so until it was white and limp. I wanted to keep it connected just a little while longer but the cord started to feel cold and I wondered if my baby could sense the change of temperature.

We tied off with a cord tie I braided and sterilized a razor blade to cut the cord. Once she was separated from her placenta we cuddled with big sister Kami and watched Teen Titans Go on the laptop. Uncle Manny and the kids were still at the hotel so we waited for them to come home. When the kids made it home they were so excited to meet their new baby sister! They pushed on my tummy to feel how soft it was and gave me and baby hugs and kisses. Such a sweet moment. They were so accepting of a new addition to the household.

The rest is pure bliss!

We have power now. The island is slowly recovering.

Accessing Her Inner Power Through Birth
Submitted by Haley Brianna Wolf

MARCH 15TH, 2018

I started having lower back cramps, intense pressure and cervical twinges throughout the day. These same sensations that I had been feeling for weeks before now felt more "real." I just intuitively knew that labor would begin within the next day.

While putting my son Asher to bed that night, I started feeling actual surges in my lower back. They grew stronger and became more frequent later that night while Tyson and I played a card game. They were still mild, but were definitely not just "practice contractions." We finally decided to go to bed at 1 a.m. so we could rest before the big event. I joked that I was too excited to sleep. The joke was on me because they quickly became too intense to sleep through!

By 4 a.m., I was needing to breathe through the waves and repeat, "Open… open…." At around 4:20, I texted my mom that I would probably need her today, as her job was to watch Asher. I went back to the bed.

At 5 a.m., I got up again as they were too strong when lying down. I spent time in the living room going through the rushes, reading my birth affirmations aloud. For the first time since painting my affirmations, I was experiencing their power. At 5:30, I told my mom to pick up a few things when the stores open and to come over as soon as possible since the drive is 40 minutes.

Only 10 minutes later, I heard Asher wake up. I got my partner, Tyson, up too and told him my mom was coming soon. "So should I go to work?" Tyson asked, still half asleep. "No, you are not going to work!" I laughed, surprised that he even asked.

I continued flowing with the waves in my birth space. "Open... open...open..." By 7:30, my waves had grown intense, but I was so exhausted from not sleeping. I knew I didn't have the strength to birth like this, so I went to have a nap. I was terrified to lie down because I feel overpowered by birth sensations in that position. My body must have known it was necessary because the frequency of surges slowed down the second I got in the bed.

I woke up a couple hours later to my mom having arrived. The frequency of my surges picked up immediately after getting out of bed, but then decreased again due to my mom and Asher being there. I wasn't able to be in the proper head space and I felt like my physical birth space was not yet mine to claim.

As I was getting Asher ready on the floor, I had an incredibly forceful surge that I nearly couldn't breathe through! I knew this was it. My mom and Asher left right away at 10:30 a.m. The following waves continued to pick up more and more in intensity. Tyson started filling up the birth pool with water.

Unlike my first birth, where I was mostly quiet and "Zen," I now needed to start vocalizing to get through. I started out self-conscious, restricting what I allowed to come out. After a couple surges of this, I reminded myself that I was a wild birthing warrior and any uncomfortable feelings did not serve me and were not mine. After that, I let go of my need to control and allowed my vocalizations to come out to meet the intensity of the sensations I was experiencing.

The sensations felt totally different from those of my birth with Asher, (which was exclusively back labor). These ones felt like a thick burning ring all the way around my pelvic area, pushing down through my cervix and vagina, and even out my urethra. I texted Jaime, my Doula, "I don't remember there being so much pressure so early and feeling like the baby was already coming down." What I really wanted to say was, "I feel that I'm really close," but I was also thinking that I'd barely been in active labor long at all- of course I wasn't close! Jaime had a mandatory meeting for her practicum that day from 9 a.m. to 2 p.m., which is why I hadn't told her to come over.

In my birth space, (which I never fully finished setting up in early labor), I would pace in circles, vocalize, and read my affirmations. The affirmations were the only thing helping me through the waves. One painting that I'd done said, "I am a warrior goddess! I AM Powerful! I AM Fearless!"

I declared out loud, "I am powerful!", and just like many times throughout my pregnancy, I automatically began to cry when saying those words. Until a few months leading up to the birth, I had never said those words. I had never believed them. Now I knew I had my power deep down inside, waiting for me to claim it. But just like nearly all women, I'd been conditioned to suppress and disconnect from it. After declaring my power, I felt a boost of confidence. Today would be the first day that I'd access it.

After about 30 minutes, I began to feel that I was losing my ability to cope with each surge. I was trying to hold myself on various things around the house, but I always felt like everything was too low to the ground. I couldn't be on my knees and leaning over too much also made me feel like I had less control. The burning in my lower back was so strong! Also unlike my first birth, counter-pressure from Tyson was not helping my back. I felt helpless, like there was nothing Tyson could do to help me. Finally, I was able to find relief with a hot compress.

I had one surge that overcame me. As I felt the surge intensifying, I heard and saw a bird hit the window. Shock. I immediately felt my body tighten more fiercely than it previously had. I dropped down to the floor, wriggling in pain, completely unable to access the proper headspace. Tyson, who was still filling the pool, ran to my side. This is when I knew I needed to find a pattern and find my power immediately.

I realized that the waves were crashing down on me, overpowering me. Reading my favorite affirmation aloud, "I release and flow with the power of my surges," I was reminded that instead of fighting my way through the waves, I needed to ride along with them. They and my baby were taking me on a journey and my job was to relax and allow the process to move through my body.

I was determined to stay above the waves. I felt the next wave about to begin. While circling in my space, I repeated, "I'm riding the waves… riding… riding the waves….” I was visualizing myself staying above them. I felt myself glide and hover over the pain. I was doing it! After the climax, I realized the power that I had accessed and uncontrollably started to cry. I continued to repeat my mantra as the wave tapered off. For the very first time, I had truly stepped in to my true power. The power that all women hold deep down and have wired in to us, but dampened and lost in the conditioning of our society. That power was beyond words. A breakthrough.

I continued this pattern throughout the remainder of my waves. Each one grew more and more in intensity. My vocalization grew fiercer to combat the intensity of the surges, keeping me level with the wave. Louder, harder, less reserved. Wild. Just when it would be about to crash over me, I would repeat, "Ride the wave, I'm riding the wave…." The power I accessed on top of each wave was just as monumental as the last. I couldn't process all of my newfound power and it would pour over in tears. I would continue with vocalizing or saying, "Open…" until the wave would dissipate.

By now, the hot compress was a crutch. I needed it HOT! Without it, there was panic. I should have known I was nearing the end! The surges were coming one after another. I couldn't tell where one ended and the next began. Spiraling around the room, almost screaming at the sensations now, I would exasperate, "Riding… I'm riding…", and just when I felt like I wouldn't be able to cope any longer, I felt a satisfying pop and warm gush of fluid down my leg. My waters breaking felt like such a relief! I ripped my underwear off and called Tyson over.

The birth pool still wasn't full. That was fine. I was never sure about whether I would birth in the pool or not anyway, and I had needed to be walking around freely during the waves. Unsure if the surges would continue with more intensity, I told Tyson to call Jaime. I was terrified of it getting any stronger. She said she would ask to leave the mandatory meeting she was at early and head over right away. Considering we live 40 minutes out of the city, I didn't think she would arrive before the baby!

It had been about 5 minutes since my water broke and still no surges. It was such a needed break! I couldn't tell if I had to poop or if it was the baby coming down. I promised myself I wouldn't give birth in the bathroom (I really envisioned my baby being born in my beautiful birth space or in our bed), but guess where it happened? Yep, the bathroom! I relocated to the bathroom in case I had to go. The pressure was definitely from the baby.

It had been about 10-15 minutes when the surges picked up again. When the first one began, I was really drawn to lean over the bathtub. Tyson's job now was to hold the hot washcloth on my back and make sure to reheat it between sensations. I got him to bring a big couch pillow for my knees.

During my entire pregnancy, I was so positive that I would not want to check my dilation whatsoever during (or before) the birth process. But in the moment, I found myself needing to be sure of whether these were a continuation of the previous surges or if the baby had begun their descent. Checking myself, way at the top of the birth canal I felt my baby! It was amazing! In an instant, I felt rejuvenated. I turned to Tyson and exclaimed almost in tears, "Oh my god! We're doing it! We're actually doing it!" Tyson sounded just as amazed and ecstatic as I was. I will cherish this moment forever.

I was very confident in my decision to birth "unassisted" from the beginning, but this was the first time I truly knew I could do it on this level. It went from an idea to a powerful and surreal reality! I felt it so deeply in my core. After the next surge, I checked myself again and I no longer felt the baby. For a moment I felt disappointment. Maybe I didn't actually feel the baby the first time? But sure enough, the baby was there again after the following rush! Wave after wave, this pattern repeated; the baby would descend during the surge and ascend during the break. I never stopped checking the baby's position during breaks. My baby and my body; working perfectly, intuitively, harmoniously. Stretching my body slowly and gently. Our bodies and babies are so smart.

Knowing that I needed to open my pelvis, I raised my right knee and shifted my weight forward and back in lunge-like motions. I had it in my mind that I wasn't going to push at all and just allow the fetal ejection reflex to take over when ready, but the sensations were so intense and I was feeling worn out. Now, in the reality of it, I would push briefly at times during surges when I felt intuitively that it was okay to do so.

Each surge was growing much more intense! My intuitive vocalization was at some points turning in to yelling. I hadn't had long enough breaks in the past hours for bits of food or drinks. I was exhausted and needed to refuel.

I found some much needed relief by sitting on the toilet. After pushing during a few surges on the toilet, the baby was sitting about half way down the birth canal. Now I needed to stand with my right leg lifted up on the bathtub's ledge with each surge. My left arm, with a casted broken wrist, was now supporting the rest of my weight on the bathroom counter. At this point I was actively pushing. During breaks, Tyson would very quickly give me sips of water, coconut water, and a bite of fruit. It had been an hour since my water broke.

I was exhausted, I felt ravaged. As a surge would begin, I would shoot up off the toilet in to position. As it would cease, I'd collapse back on the toilet, needing fuel to give me energy for the next wave. I would check the baby towards the end of each rush. It was so very close to crowning each time! At the end, I would feel the baby move back up.

Just then, I heard Jaime walk in the door! She came in and asked if I'd like her to take photos. Of course! (I am so beyond grateful for her divine timing. I got my intimate birth experience with my partner, alone, and also got the most incredible pictures of our final, and our baby's first moments!)

Now I was no longer sitting back on the toilet. I was hovering during breaks, my leg on the bath, casted arm on the counter. Tyson and I were staring in to each other's eyes, waiting for the next wave.

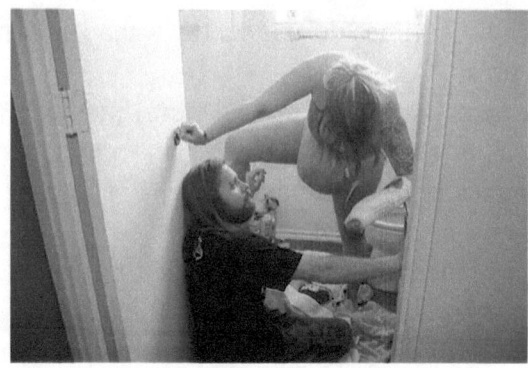

I knew in all my being that this had to be it.

With this rush, I pushed with all my strength. I felt the baby's head coming through! It moved back up slightly, but I could still feel the head of hair right there at the opening during the break. With the next rush I pushed, breathed, pushed, breathed, and intuitively listening to my body. My hand feeling my tissue slowly stretch paper thin and open. Burning! Crowning, I felt the baby's head lock in to place! I now remembered the feeling of the "ring of fire," although I would describe it as pressure.

During this pause, I just soaked in this magic between worlds. Feeling how thin my tissues had stretched, feeling the wet hair on my baby's head, waiting in this openness. Knowing that any SECOND I would be meeting this person that Tyson and I called in. This person who I had grown in my body for 43 weeks. There are no words.

Here it was, the final surge. I pushed again with all my strength! I felt the baby's head sliding through… Wait… Breathe, push… Breathe, okay puuush—I felt the baby's head pop out (with a hand at his face)! RELIEF!

Within the next second, my hand still holding the head, I guided my baby out in to my partner's loving arms as the rest of the body shot out. I DID IT! I felt power and strength that I still haven't found the words to describe. I looked down and was shocked to see a boy! We had been expecting a girl from very early on. Tyson and I looked at each other with confused faces. Jaime said our look was priceless! He cried as he was still coming out of my body and had amazing color already. Tyson swears he heard the name Zephyr within seconds of seeing our boy. I believe him completely.

Zephyr Nova was born on March 16th, 2018 at *approximately* 2:13 p.m. at 42+6 weeks.

I had an intact perineum. No tearing whatsoever! Jaime helped us move effortlessly to the bedroom. I delivered my placenta spontaneously in the comfort of my bed within 30 minutes of birth. For me it's relevant to add that being at home, I had no one pushing on my uterus after birth while trying to bond with my baby. It did its job, which it's obviously made to do. I was able to feel it and decide for myself if it was contracting properly. To me, the pain of the uterine "massage" post birth was significantly more painful than the entire birth process. No one prepared me for it either. I feel like I still hold trauma from that in my hospital birth with Asher.

We were able to instinctively navigate the immediate postpartum, with all the hormones working harmoniously in our favor. Just like nature intended. Even with only one hand, breastfeeding was a breeze. I had no one telling me what to do, telling me that I needed to track my baby. No one testing my baby and taking him away. Since I never got to use my birth pool, I washed off in it a couple hours postpartum. We did a cord burning ceremony after I asked Zephyr if it was okay for me to separate him from his placenta so that I could consume it. He didn't cry so I took it as a yes. He also didn't cry during the separation. After the cord burning, my mom brought Asher home and he got to meet his baby brother!

I, (or should I say we), had a placenta smoothie. Tyson was already open to trying it, Asher had a couple cups, and even my mom who was wary about the thought earlier became curious and had a few sips! We weighed him late that night. He was 7.7 lbs. Both having no routine prenatal care and birthing undisturbed and free have been the most rewarding experiences of my life!

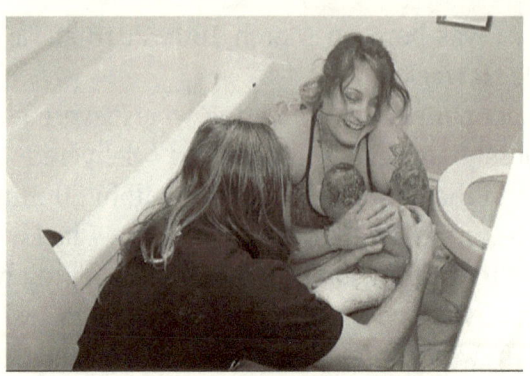

You can follow Haley and find out more about her transformational healing program for women on her website. www.firewithinbirthfreedom.com

VBAC/HBAC Freebirths

An Ode to Fearless Women

Defined by no man, you are your own story, blazing
through the world, turning history into herstory.
And when they dare to tell you about all the things you
cannot be,
you smile and tell them, "I am both war and woman
and you cannot stop me."

- poem by Nikita Gill

The Birth of Mordekai: Our En Caul Experience
Submitted by Michelle Huddleston

THE JOURNEY STARTED EARLY spring with a faint-positive pregnancy test, and yet another surprise from Abba. My husband and I had mutually agreed that we would not prevent conception, although we are not planning either. It's funny to see people's faces when they ask how many children we plan on having, and we respond with however many God blesses us with!

From the conception of our daughter five years ago, our research to all-natural births started. This took us down the path to everything from home births and midwives to natural remedies and Doulas (and everything in between). We are forever grateful for this journey because with each pregnancy, labor, and birth – it gets better and better! Not to mention, our faith grows stronger and stronger!

Most people in our neck of the Kentucky woods think we are crazy. Others think we are being irresponsible. And there are those who actually express their deep desire in wanting to experience a natural childbirth, but couldn't for whatever reason. Regardless of what others think, we know that our choice to do home births is for us. Our choice to have an educated, unassisted pregnancy and home birth is for us.

Yes, you read that right… an educated, unassisted pregnancy and home birth. It is not for everyone. Without going down the path of stating the obvious, there are many reasons why some women have to utilize modern medicine care (regardless of the reason), and that's okay. You will not read any mom-shaming here. Quite frankly, this isn't about anyone else but our family, and our choice to birth how we see fit.

Okay.... at this point you are probably wondering, "so how did the birth of Mordekai go?" It went like this....

Braxton Hick's contractions were my best friend since the second trimester. They were nothing new and I knew they were prepping my body for the grand finale. As weeks went on, my body definitely showed it's age (thirty-something), but I attempted to embrace that as well. I must admit that I didn't workout near as much as past pregnancies, and I actually enjoyed my late night cookies and milk snacks.

As the due date of December 4th approached, I grew more and more anxious at the thought of my bundle arriving "early, as expected, or late." You see, my first born was a planned induction (I will NEVER do that again) at 38 weeks.... our daughter was a successful home birth at 40+2 and actually ended in a transport that resulted in a D&C to get the rest of the placenta out that caused PPH (too much midwife intervention).... and our second son was a successful and perfect unassisted home birth at 39 weeks (the midwife didn't make it to the birth in time).

With Mordekai (sex unknown at the time), 39 weeks came and went. Then 40 weeks. It was 7-ish in the morning on Monday, December 4th (2017) when I started having contractions that seemed to stick around. Not like the prodromal labor I experienced last pregnancy, but more like the progressing "real thing" that I experienced with our daughter. One after the other, I was convinced that this would be the day that we would finally meet our baby.

I attempted to go about the day as normal but finally told my husband that I needed to be able to just labor. Instantly, he kicks into super Dad mode and takes over the kiddos. They were surprisingly AMAZING at watching me labor (as I needed Daddy to squeeze my hips with each contraction as they grew stronger). They took turns rubbing my back and talking to me, although my oldest (10 year old) was a little shocked and partly upset that he couldn't understand the pain.

As contractions progressed, it actually worked perfectly because as I approached transition, the kiddos were laying down for their naps. At this time, it's about 11ish a.m. and I had been relaxing and riding the waves in a bathtub full of warm water for about 30 minutes. This helped ease the contractions some, but I looked at my husband and told him to get the pillows and towels because I was getting out of the bathtub. In my mind, I was determined to start riding these waves with the thought of meeting our bundle sooner rather than later. In other words…I was going to start pushing.

And I did.

The next wave came and I totally relaxed everything and "beared down" as most would say. From there, it was the point of no return. The next wave sent me into an army crawl position (which is funny because afterward, my husband asked where I was going). Then back up on all fours I went with another couple of waves and pushes. That's when Dr. Dad said he could see the baby coming and "it" (at the time we didn't know gender) appeared to still be en caul. He tried to break the bag then but couldn't get a grip. I reached back and instantly realized how slippery, but tough the sac actually was. I got a good grip of baby's head and pulled while pushing the baby out into Daddy's arms. By the time his body was out, the sac tore open.

"IT'S A BOY!!!" Bryan cried out. I sat back in instant relief and started to enjoy the fact that we just had our bundle of joy. Lots of questions went through my head about his color (which was normal), his size (which was normal), his lack of instant crying (which was normal), and so on…. but Bryan reassured me that everything was okay and went to get the things we needed to finish up (umbilical cord ring, scissors, bowl, etc.).

While waiting for the umbilical cord to stop pulsing, baby and I hopped back in the bathtub to relax and start the process of nursing. At this point, I was incredibly relieved but still knew that I had to deliver the placenta… which is something we had not done by ourselves before (yet). Sure enough, by the time the cord stopped pulsing and we got the ring on his umbilical cord, it was time to push again. I delivered the placenta with grace and ease into a bowl and felt even better.

The rest of the story consists of a shower, freshening up, and basking in the fact that we just finished up an educated, unassisted pregnancy and home birth!

It's amazing how our bodies know exactly what to do. They are truly designed and made to function in ways that far exceed anything that can be understood at times, and I'm thankful for trusting YHVH to guide us during such an incredible experience.

It took us a few days to finally decide on a name and get stats, but here they are: Mordekia was born at 11:25 a.m. weighing in a 7.4 lbs (my biggest baby yet) and 20" long.

Michelle doesn't claim to be a professional or anything, but what she does have is passion and the desire to see women live unapologetically authentic. If you are looking for encouragement on your mommy journey, especially for home birthing, contact her on Facebook or through her Blog. You will also find a good post or two about home births, pregnancy health, and the like.

Facebook: www.facebook.com/withthehuddlestons

Blog: https://withthehuddlestons.com

Freebirth in Autumn

Submitted by Beautiful Dunn

AUTUMN EMBER
North Dakota
Thanksgiving Day, 2016

Our first experience becoming parents was awful. It was a terrible hospital birth with no control and lies. It was a 'medical procedure', and our wishes were ignored and mocked. It ended in an unnecessary Cesarean Section, and I knew I would never give birth in a hospital again. Our second child was a completely unassisted pregnancy and birth resulting in a 9lb baby boy being born in our bathroom on Valentine's Day. It was rough, and resulted in a transfer for my care, but we were all fine.

Living in North Dakota, there isn't a lot of support for free birthing mamas, and I don't know a single person who lives here who has done it besides me. We knew all our future babies would be free births. When we found out we were expecting #3, we were overjoyed at the thought of another stress free pregnancy and powerful free birth in our home. During my pregnancy, I had a reoccurring dream of my husband coming home early in the morning while it was still dark outside, a light dusting of fresh snow falling, to find me in labor in the hallway of our home. Moments later, seeing daddy holding our baby girl in his arms even though we didn't know the baby's gender.

It was so peaceful and magical. Baby was sharing a dream with me and only me. It was our perfect birth and our bond. On Thanksgiving morning (11-24-2016) around 6:20 a.m. I was suddenly woken up and needed to use the bathroom. I went back to bed and tried to get some more sleep since my alarm would be going off in an hour so I could get ready for a 45-minute drive to a family lunch.

A few minutes later, I was woken again by some mild cramping. I glanced at the clock and noticed it was 6:28 a.m. I noted to myself my husband would be getting off work in a half hour. I then had another surge of cramping and glanced at the clock again, it was 6:30 a.m. I decided to just lay in bed and keep an eye on the clock for a little while. After another couple contractions, they began to increase in pressure, and I found myself moaning through them and talking to baby. I got out of bed and made my way to the living room, rubbing my belly and breathing deeply and calmly.

Contractions were still coming every 2-3 minutes and lasting about a minute long, but they weren't painful, just smooth waves. By this time it was close to 7 a.m., and I knew my husband, Clayton, would be getting off from work now and coming home. I looked out the window, it was still dark and very foggy, looked as if snow was falling. I felt so at peace, it felt so familiar. I smiled, knowing this is what my mind and body had been preparing for. Contractions were growing in strength and I knew if I called my hubby he would rush home and I didn't want him to get into an accident. I was resting my head on a pillow as I was bent over the bathroom sink, swaying my hips with each strong wave. I was moaning and swaying as I heard the front door open and my husband come up the stairs.

It was about 7:20 a.m., and he opened the bathroom door with a smile and said "Hey…are you in labor?" All I could do was nod my head as another contraction came, and that's when I realized this was real labor. This was it. He waited patiently in the hallway for the contraction to pass and then asked me what I needed him to do. I told him to grab me a Powerade and start filling the birth pool. I was so relieved that he was home and there for me. Contractions were coming every 1.5-2 minutes now and lasting a little over a minute long, but I continued to breathe and sway through them. My legs were getting tired, so I listened to my body and got on my hands and knees in the living room.

They kept getting more intense, and I started to loudly moan. Clayton asked if I was okay, I said I was but they were starting to get a little painful. He had aired up the pool and had just started to fill it as I thought to myself "What is he doing in there? Why is it taking him so long to get that pool ready!?" I checked the clock and felt like I had been in labor for hours but it was only 7:40 a.m.

I needed to use the bathroom again, so I made my way there. I was on the toilet for two contractions and felt uneasy, so I stood up next to the sink again. At the peak of the next contraction I felt the need to bear down and squat. I could feel the Earth beneath my feet pulling my belly down, like I couldn't control it. They were coming closer and closer, and I called for my husband. I told him there was a lot of pressure, and I needed to get on the floor. He helped me lower down and as soon as my knees hit the floor I felt intense pressure, and my water broke. It didn't just break, but it exploded out onto the towel I had on the floor. I laughed because it surprised me. I immediately felt my body start to push.

I was worried at first because I didn't think I wasn't dilated enough yet. I told Clayton I was getting that push urge, and it was too soon. I told him I couldn't keep doing it if it was going to be this intense for so long. I called out, "Please, God, don't make this last too much longer." Clayton told me to breathe, close my eyes and listen to my body. He was right, I felt panic in my mind but calm in my heart. He asked me if I wanted him to check if he could feel the baby yet. I said yes, and as soon as he checked me he happily said, "I can feel something hard, I think it's the baby's head!" I was in denial. I asked if he was sure. He said he was and that baby was coming. I was tired and wanted a break to clear my mind. Clayton told me I was doing great and that I was so strong. He told me to breathe and trust my body, that I was doing everything perfectly. It's like his words instilled some sort of confidence in me because my next words were, "I can do this. I can do this. We can do this, baby. It's me and you. We can do this."

I was squatting as I had another hard contraction. I growled and moaned deep and loud. I didn't push at all. My feet felt like they had roots firmly planted in the floor, like my body was a mighty oak that spent years growing right there, waiting for this moment to support me. Clayton said, "It's the baby's head. It's coming out!" I reached down and could feel baby's head, feel the hair. I was so relieved that this was happening so fast. I told Clayton to grab a warm washcloth, and he held it against my bottom as another strong contraction came and my body pushed on its own.

Clayton touched my back and said, "The head is out. I can see the head!" I asked if the whole head was out, mouth and nose and if baby looked okay. He smiled and said, "Yes, her lips are moving!" I didn't even have time to notice that he said "her lips," since we didn't know the gender of baby, and we already had 2 boys. My body took a short break. Clayton and I talked and laughed about how crazy this all was and that it was finally time to meet baby. About two minutes later, I felt another contraction. I told Clayton to get ready to catch baby as he sat behind me. My body pushed as I roared, and the baby slid right out into daddy's arms.

Clayton yelled, "It's a girl, we have a girl!" as he fought back tears. He held her as I turned around and sat down. I had seen this image in my dreams so many times but actually seeing it with my eyes happening right in front of me was nothing short of the most incredible moment in my life.

My husband was a little concerned, since she wasn't making any sounds. I told him it was okay, but he could rub her back a little bit if he wanted. She started to moan, and he looked at me like he never had before. So intense, so lost for words. There she was, our little Autumn Ember. I asked Clayton what time she was born. He said 8:08 a.m. It all happened in just 1 hour and 40 minutes!

Clayton handed her to me and I said I felt like I had to push again. Terror hit his face as he said, "It better not be another baby!" but I assured him it was just the placenta. Autumn was so content and just snuggled me as I burst into tears. Clayton and I sat on the bathroom floor in shock, crying together for over ten minutes. It had all been so perfect and so fast. He kissed me and that kiss somehow felt different, felt new. We felt different, the whole world felt new.

We left her cord and placenta attached for about an hour while her older brothers got to meet her. We then weighed and measured her: 9 lbs 8 oz and 20.25 inches long. We had a lot to be thankful for that Thanksgiving Day. Looking back, it's so surreal how accurate my dreams were. My body waited until baby was ready, and until I had support from my husband. It really was a dream come true. We are now 24 weeks pregnant with baby #4 and due in March of 2019. This will be our third freebirth VBAC/HBAC baby, and we are so excited to see the journey this baby takes us on.

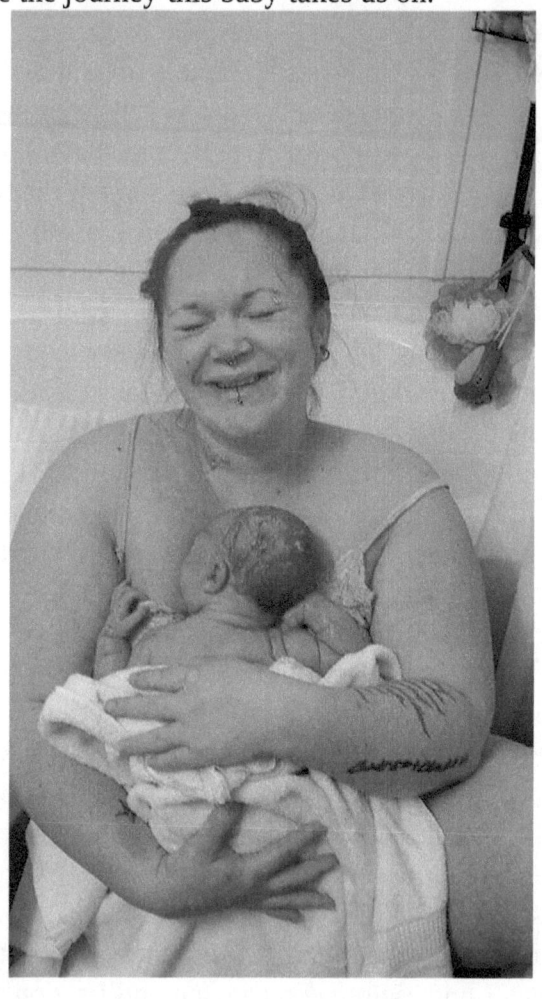

3 FBAC of Angel Finley Dunn
Submitted by Beautiful Dunn

MY GUT HAD BEEN telling me baby would come around 3-5 days after my due date. My gut also told me baby would be 10 lbs and a girl. My gut was WAY off this time.

Thursday, March 7th started as a chaotic day as it was two days before my estimated due date with baby #4 and I still had a lot to do. I took a bath and joked with baby saying that he/she could come whenever since there was no way I was getting everything done, that he/she could come that very day if that's what they wanted. I had surrendered. I then made a grocery list, started putting all my labor and birth supplies into a pile and made a plan for how to rearrange all the car seats in the car.

It was freezing outside and took me an hour and a half to get the car seats installed. I was getting lunch ready for the kids and had just put a pizza in the oven for myself because I was starving. It was around 1:30 p.m. and I just felt weird, figured I was hungry and stressed from everything I still had to do. I pulled the pizza out of the oven at 1:45 p.m. and felt a surge of pressure in my hips. I brushed it off and 2 minutes later, there was another. I figured it was early labor or prodromal as they were not painful and all my babies had come a few days after due date, never before.

I kept ignoring them but texted my husband that I was having some contractions. He asked if it was labor, I said no. Then at 2:00 p.m., I found myself leaning over the bathroom sink moaning. I texted him again saying they were getting stronger and I was moaning through them. He called me and asked if I needed him home, I said "No, I don't know how long this will last and you only have an hour left."

He ignored my words and said he would be on his way. As soon as I hung up, they were coming every minute and were lasting almost 2 minutes long while I sat backwards on the toilet. The kids (ages 5, 4 and 2) would come check on me when they heard me moan. They would kiss me or rub my back saying, "It's ok, mommy." It was nice having them there to support me. At 2:20 p.m., I started to feel heat in my thighs during the contractions. They were getting somewhat painful but I tried to envision baby coming down with each wave. At 2:25 p.m., I heard my husband come through the door and up the stairs to the bathroom.

He asked how I was doing but I couldn't talk as the contractions were back to back and not letting up. My 2 year old daughter came in and gave me a kiss and asked, "is baby hurting your gina?" I told her yes but that baby was coming soon. She kissed me and left as I started feeling FER kick in. I started having intense pressure building and building with my body pushing hard. I reached down to feel the sack bulging.

I told my husband I could feel the amniotic sack, and he asked if I could get off the toilet so he could help me. I couldn't move as another strong contraction started and FER pushed again. This time the sack exploded into the toilet as I reached down to feel it. Without a break, FER continued to push as I felt the head start to emerge. It didn't stop until the head was completely out and I shouted, "it's the head, I'm holding the head, the head is out!"

My husband told me to get up so he could help catch, knowing I have short arms and wouldn't be able to catch baby myself. I held the head as I stood up and took one step back. I dropped to one knee and another contraction came, pushing the body out with another huge explosion of water. My husband caught the baby and shouted "it's a boy, we have another boy!"

My phone was sitting in front of me and said 2:42 p.m. The whole labor from first contraction to baby born was 57 minutes, a new record for me! I turned around and my husband handed the baby to me. He was crying a little bit but stopped as soon as I held him. He seemed so tiny compared to the others (8lb 4oz, 20" long). I could tell I tore by how forceful FER had been, but I wasn't sore at all. A couple minutes later, the placenta came out and was so small compared to the others too.

The cord was very short (13.5"), so I had to keep the bowl with the placenta on my lap just to hold baby. He started nursing right away and after an hour, we got cleaned up. The kids trailed in one by one to welcome their little brother Ansel Finley Dunn and give him a kiss. It had all started, happened and ended so fast! Our third completely unassisted home birth after a c-section. We were now a family of 6 with 3 boys and 1 girl. Even though so much had changed, it felt the same as it ever did.

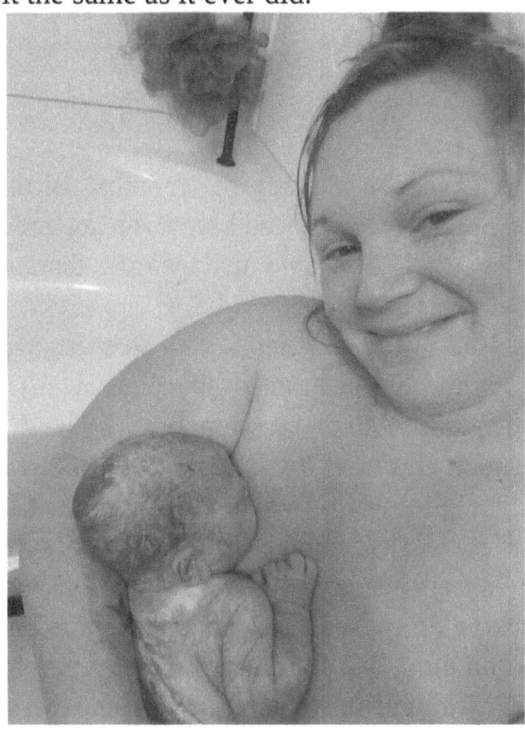

Anniversary Surprise

Submitted by Haley

FINLEY

South Carolina, U.S.A.

My birth space had been ready for months. Birth affirmations, tinctures, everything we would need before during and after the birth was ready. I knew my baby would arrive earlier than my due date, it was just a matter of when.

We woke up Halloween morning with a stomach virus. It fiercely took over our entire day and ruined any plans we had for trick or treating with the kids. All of us were sick. I knew I was getting dehydrated by noon and tried my hardest to keep any type of liquid down to avoid going into labor while still so sick and weak. That did not work. I was 37 weeks pregnant, and it was baby time. We spent the entire day in bed just trying to rest. The day was a blur, and finally the throwing up ceased and everyone went to bed.

My labor began around 2 a.m. the following morning, November 1st. I tossed and turned most of the night, and began waking up every few minutes to painful contractions. Around 3 a.m. I had to get out of bed. Nothing could keep me still, I needed to move. I paced around stopping for contractions and grabbing onto the nearest hard surface to sway through the surges. I still wasn't convinced this was true labor because I'd been experiencing prodromal labor for over a month at this point. I assumed the dehydration from throwing up most of the day was causing my contractions to pick up, but that with some rest and water they would subside. I decided to shower and see if that slowed anything down. I know I showered, because my hair was wet the rest of that morning, but I honestly barely even remember it. I think my time in the shower was for me to go away to "labor land" and get ready for what was coming.

Once 4 a.m. came along, I started to realize the contractions were only getting stronger and closer together, so I went to the bed and nudged my husband Jamie. "I don't wanna do this alone anymore." He knew before falling asleep I was having some more intense contractions, so he was aware that things were getting serious now. He shot right out of bed and followed me through our bedroom and bathroom as I dealt with each contraction.

The stronger they got, the louder I got, and I needed his support to stand through them. I remember being surprised with how loud I felt like I needed to be, roaring through every surge. I always imagined myself to be quiet and reserved during natural labor, but there was no way around it; I had to be vocal. I remember being somewhat vocal with my first two births, laboring to 10 cm naturally both times. But this time was different. I had so much back labor now. I found out later that was because Finley was sunny-side-up until I'm assuming crowning. I was also so weak and tired from the sickness the day before.

Jamie began pushing on my lower back at my request, which helped ease the pain for a short time as I neared transition. I'm not sure how much time passed by, but I remember feeling weak from not eating most of the day, and really wanting to get in the bath. Jamie started it for me, steam pouring over the edges of our tub. Every now and then I was checking myself, searching for my baby's head in hopes the end was near. This time, there was some bloody show. Oddly enough, that is when it hit me. This was real. I was meeting my baby today. I looked at the red on my fingers and realized how insanely amazing this was. I was in labor about to have my baby. No one was making this happen. No one was telling me where to go or what to do. Just me and my body working to bring my child earth-side. I didn't need any help. I could do this.

Once I got in the water, things really picked up. They say water can boost labor sometimes, and that was very true in my case. I slowly started to feel small urges to push, which I held back as best as I could, knowing I would need to rest in the bath while I still had the chance. I think this was the point in labor where I felt like I was screaming through every contraction. Jamie later told me that I was not nearly as loud as I thought I was, but I felt like the entire neighborhood could hear me! I leaned over the tub on my knees as another surge came. There was a very loud and shocking splash. My first thought was, "Oh my god, my baby just fell out!", but of course that was the delusion of dehydration and exhaustion speaking.

"Holy cow was that your water breaking?!" Jamie asked. And it was. I only knew then because of the intensity the end of that contraction had. I thought I might faint. I needed out of the tub right then and there, so I stood up and we laid out towels and Chux pads in the bedroom floor and shut off all the lights. My baby was coming! Jamie got the birthing ball for me which I am so grateful for because at the time I didn't think I wanted it at all. Apparently, he knew better. I shifted from my hands and knees to hanging my arms over the ball with my knees on the floor. The urge to push was impossible to fight now. I couldn't stop my body from pushing, the urge was deep and primal.

I soon felt the burning that could only mean my baby was crowning! Contractions couldn't have been more than 30 seconds apart at this point, and I can remember only wanting a tiny break, just a moment to ground myself. I kept saying "I just want to lay down for a minute." But it was too uncomfortable to lie flat. I tried lying on our bed and immediately stood back up with the next surge. As the burning got worse, I reached to feel for baby's head again. I looked at Jamie with a weak smile and said, "I can feel his hair!" The smile faded as I started to believe there was no way I could get this baby out, but my body continued to push. I wanted to fight the pushing because of the burning, but I couldn't stop. He was coming down so incredibly fast without me even trying to push. I told Jamie, "He is NOT going to fit, get me a mirror!" He did. I took my first look at what was going on down there and said quietly, "Okay, maybe he is fitting," as I realized most of his head was out. I couldn't believe this. I was doing it! My body was doing this all on its own.

My baby was close, and I knew with the next few pushes his head would be out! Two more surges and then pure relief as his head escaped. There is no relief in the world like that feeling. I felt like I could do anything in that moment. My body gave me a brief break as Finley rested between two worlds. I could feel him wiggling, turning himself and getting ready for his hasty exit. I told Jamie to get behind me and get ready to catch as another urge to push neared. Another two surges and I felt him fall out of me and into his daddy's hands.

"Oh! It's a boy!" I heard him almost laugh. I turned around and sat down so I could hold this beautiful brand-new creature, and I kept saying over and over, "Oh, hello baby, hi sweet boy!" I couldn't believe I'd done it. And I was holding my precious little boy in my arms, the very first time ever delivering and being able to immediately hold my child. There are no words to describe how fulfilling that moment was. I was beaming, in another world of pure magic. It was 6:30 a.m. at this point. We quickly walked back to the bathroom, and I got in the tub while we waited for the placenta to deliver, which came only a few short minutes later. I noticed shortly after that, that his cord had a true knot in it, which is supposed to be good luck. I felt his cord and stared at it and the placenta, amazed at the beauty of this life-sustaining organ. Jamie looked at me and said, "Happy anniversary." I realized it was indeed our anniversary. What a special gift for us to share together after four years of marriage.

Once the cord stopped pulsing, Jamie went downstairs to boil the scissors and cord tie we had made with our oldest two children, and brought them back up to me. He also let Jayce into our bedroom, who had just woken up to the sounds of his baby brother crying. Jayce laid in our bed, waiting to meet his new brother, still quite tired from the day before. Jamie tied, and I cut the cord myself. We wrapped Finley up in a towel, and I nursed him for the first time. I passed Finley to his daddy and took a quick shower to gather my wits and clean up a bit.

When I came back into the bedroom, I pointed to Finley and asked Jayce, "Who is this?" He smiled and said "Poppy Seed!" which was this surprise gender baby's nickname while he lived in me. We told Jayce it was a boy, and he was over the moon. Lilly joined us soon after, met our newest addition, and soon she and Jayce both fell back asleep in the early morning light. The day quieted down. I took a dropper full of my Shepherd's Purse tincture and put a piece of placenta in my cheek to help slow my bleeding a little while I worked on getting Finley latched on again.

The rest of this beautiful morning was a blur of warm joy. I drifted in and out of sleep with my baby in my arms while the T.V. played quietly in the background and the kids ate their Poptarts on the bedroom floor. We talked about baby names throughout the day (we hadn't yet decided on one), and all four of us finally chose Finley William. William is my dad's middle name, and we wanted to pass it down the same way we passed Jamie's dad's middle name down to Jayce. We let our family and friends know of the wonderful news, all of whom were so proud and excited for us. One of the best parts of this experience was the love and support I had in my choices to birth free.

Although this birth was a difficult one due to illness and exhaustion before even beginning, it was the most empowering and magical experience of my life. Delivering our child at home with only each other was so perfect. Finley is the happiest and healthiest of babies, and I wouldn't trade this memory for the world. My free birth was everything I wanted it to be and more, and the healing I got from it, the bond I have with Finley, is like nothing else in the entire world.

Magic. Pure magic.

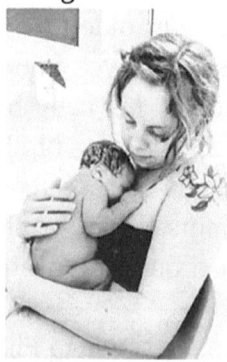 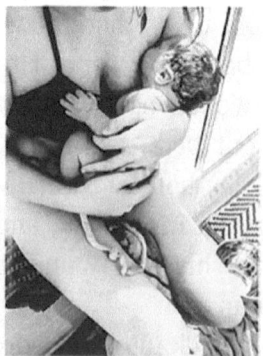

You can continue to follow Haley and her story as it unfolds on her blog: www.bloomingnewlife.com

The Breech Birth of Tobie
Submitted by Katie

REDDING, CALIFORNIA

In 2009 I gave birth to my first via a very traumatic C-section after a very long labor. My second and third babies were born at home with midwives. I can't tell you exactly why I decided to do unassisted with our fourth. I loved our Midwife from our third birth and she was still available but for some reason I was just drawn into doing it on our own. I had a Doppler so I listened to baby's heartbeat throughout the pregnancy, I checked my blood pressure on occasion but other than that I didn't do much, besides wait.

On January 24th 2018, I gave birth to my fourth boy with my third HBAC, first unassisted birth. He was our rainbow baby after an early miscarriage a year and two days before his birth. Like his three older brothers, his due date came and went with no sign of him. He was 8 days past his due date when he made his entrance.

With my last birth, my water broke a few hours before contractions so I wasn't able to ever check my cervix, which I was bummed about. This time contractions started very mildly about 6 a.m. after a very restless night with lots of cramping and lower back pain. At around seven I decided to check my cervix because I was in total denial that I was in actual labor. I had checked my cervix off and on throughout my pregnancy just to get an idea of what my normal was, and right away I could feel there was already a big difference in my cervix. I checked my cervix throughout labor and it was incredibly cool to feel the changes. After my cervix had opened quite a bit and I could feel past the cervix, I was amazed how soft baby's head felt. I assumed there must have been a lot of amniotic fluid between the baby's head and the sack. Had I not been aware how dilated I was, I'm not sure I would have realized how close he was to being born. My labor never really intensified and I never went through what felt like a transition. I could feel baby moving down the birth canal and the contractions got maybe a little bit stronger but nothing like my previous births.

Once I felt like my cervix was no longer where I could feel it and I was getting uncomfortable, I started to fill up our Jacuzzi tub in our master bath. I got in and instantly it was heavenly. By about 10 a.m. I was starting to feel the need to push and I could feel baby in the birth canal, so I pushed when it felt right. My husband was hanging out close by during pushing, and at one point said, "Wow, that's a tiny head." Once the first part of baby started coming out, I kept waiting for that relief once the head is out where it feels like baby isn't going to slide back up inside you, but that relief never came. I continued pushing until baby was about 3/4 of the way out and then my husband announced, "Oh shoot, it's feet!" Turns out baby was frank breech and he was still completely closed in the sack until he was out up to about his armpits and when his feet popped out they broke the sack. I just kept pushing because it felt right and I knew not to touch baby. Finally he popped out, did a little flip in the water and his daddy reached in, picked him up, handed him to me and said "Here's your baby!"

I kept saying I can't believe how tiny he seemed and talking to him and rubbing his back, trying to get him to perk up a little bit. He was pretty limp and other than his eyes opening, wasn't responsive or putting much effort into breathing. I know it's normal for breech babies to take a little bit to get going sometimes so I wasn't too worried the first couple minutes but after 2-3 minutes I was starting to get a little impatient for him to perk up a little more. He finally did start breathing better, let out a little cry and got some more tone to him and pinked up nicely. Once he was looking good we checked to see that we had our fourth boy. He had had a pretty good size bowel movement in the sack so there was meconium on him and in the tub. I knew to be extra diligent to make sure he hadn't inhale any.

We hung out in the bath for almost two hours waiting for the placenta to finally come out. I knew from my previous births that I wanted to nurse baby as soon as possible to help with my bleeding, so I got him latched on and he nursed away. His eyes were wide open while we were in the tub and he was looking around checking out everything. Once the placenta was delivered, we moved to the bed where we cut the cord, weighed and measured and nursed and snuggled some more. He came in at 8 lb even and 20 inches long. Almost the exact size of his two oldest Brothers but a lot smaller than his closest brother who came in at 9 lbs 15 oz 21 inches long.

We took a couple of days to decide for sure on his name, but finally decided on Tobie Malakai.

It ended up being myself, my husband, our oldest son who was 8, our 18 month old and my friend's two girls who were 11 and 13 at the birth. I had planned on catching baby myself, but then my husband jumped in and did it and I was so glad he did. We had booked a birth photographer that photographed our previous birth, but of course she was out of town the 23rd to the 25th and he came on the 24th. The 13 year old took pictures, and she did a fantastic job. I wouldn't change a single thing about this birth.

It feels pretty amazing to know that I accomplished an unassisted birth, a home birth, a water birth, a vaginal birth after a c-section and a breech birth, all in one beautiful, perfect birth.

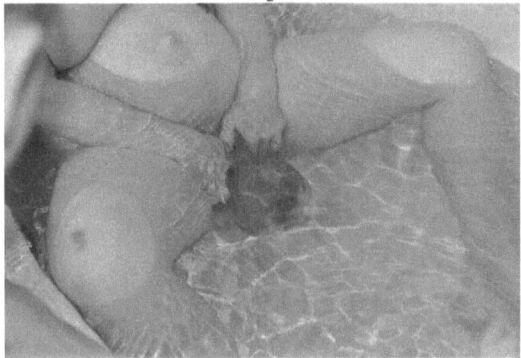

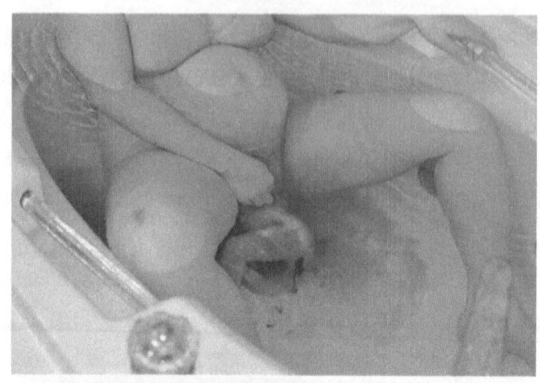
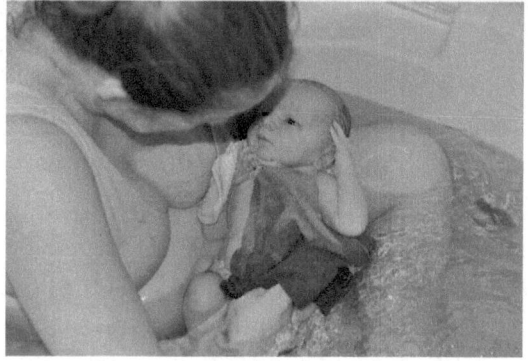

Pleasurable Freebirths

"Giving birth is a highly creative act full of orgasmic feelings, and can be a moment of ecstatic pleasure for the mother."
— *"Mental First Aid in Pregnancy and Childbirth,"
by Joost A.M. Meerloo, M.D. (Child and Family, Fall 1966)*

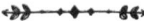

Birth Before Dinner
Submitted by Heather Bailey

CHRISTOPHER
Born January 26, 2016.
Salt Lake City, Utah

With my first birth, I prepared by taking a Hypnobabies class and hiring a Midwife at a birth center. Baby Ashley came early (5 weeks), and spent 2 weeks at the NICU (an emotional roller coaster for me being separated from my baby, but it all ended well). My baby Ashley came home on Mother's Day, a wonderful gift.

Birth #2 was quite fast, I woke up in the middle of the night (3 a.m.?) to my water breaking, took an hour to get ready. When my body began pushing, I realized we needed to get to the birth center NOW, so we got our 2-yr-old daughter into the car and rushed to the birth center. Baby Bradley was born 11 minutes after we pulled up (3-5 minutes after getting into the birthing room). We called our mothers and our Doula to let them know baby Bradley had arrived. A few hours later, we went home together as a new family.

I never thought I'd ever give birth in a restaurant, but I did. It was a planned unassisted home birth, with a surprise location.

I planned and prepared for Christopher's birth for many months. We lived up a long snowy canyon with a huge driveway up to our home, and he was due to come in mid-snowy-winter. With the present situation, and following our intuition, we felt it best to stay home for this birth (our first two were born under midwife care at a birth center). I always have amazing births, a mixture of calm, and intense, but still doable. Along with my breathing and relaxation, I have relied on my husband's positive reassurance to help me through to the end. Especially right before the birth when all the doubt hits, he's been there for me.

My amazing friend I hired as a Doula for my 2nd baby's birth (who came so fast we called our Doula after the baby's birth) had recently given birth to her 3rd child unassisted. Intrigued, I wanted to learn more from her because I am a very intuitive, internally-processing person, and I know I make better decisions with less people/influencers in the room, especially while giving birth. I felt it right in my heart to listen and learn from her and follow the same path to a successful unassisted birth for my 3rd child.

I hired her as a Doula and unassisted birth mentor to teach me all I needed to prepare for this birth. I learned who to contact for filing a birth certificate, and that I needed an official proof of pregnancy for it. She gave me different possible circumstances to research and create solutions for if things didn't go as planned. I shared my research and solutions with my husband, and he felt calm and prepared as well. We discussed and answered all our "what if" questions until we both felt peaceful about it.

A side note, I was willing to go the hospital or see a midwife if I felt I needed it, but my preference was to stay at home. I made plans/preparations for different possible outcomes, but I expected and anticipated the absolute best birth experience.

Now here's where the restaurant as the birth location comes in: We expected our baby to come right around Valentine's Day, so we planned our own celebration a few weeks early, thinking that would give us plenty of time before baby comes. An early January morning, I woke up with consistent contractions every 5-10 minutes. When I got out of bed, they stopped, and it seemed the birth could still be 1-2 weeks away. I felt it best to go about my day as planned. I took my 2 children to their music class, with contractions coming off and on (not so pleasant while sitting on the floor in class with my kids, but still manageable).

We all got home, and my husband and I planned to leave on our 3-day celebration together. Our babysitter arrived, and we left for a close-to-home getaway. I packed some baby items "just in case." We left for our first activity, a play that ended up being hilarious, and with contractions coming every so often, that made it really awkward to laugh so hard.

After the play, contractions still seemed very light and Braxton Hicks-y, so we headed over to a nice Italian restaurant. They sat us by a fireplace, very romantic, and I had Eric sit by the fire so I wouldn't feel too uncomfortably warm. With our bread plate and appetizers coming out, the contractions started getting closer and stronger. With each intense wave, I closed my eyes, held Eric's hand, and relaxed and breathed through it. These waves of contractions started coming about every 1-3 minutes. (Our server had no idea I was even having contractions because I was so relaxed and calm on the outside.)

At this point, I turned to Eric and asked, "What do we do? Should we go home, or go to a nearby hotel?" But again, we felt peaceful about staying (I was thinking birth was still hours away at least).

Right before the main course was supposed to be served, I thought "I'm not hungry, how could I eat any more food?" So, just to clear my mind, I excused myself and went to the bathroom.

After a couple minutes, I was about to go back to our table when the thought and feeling came to me to sit back down on the toilet. Immediately, as I was sitting back down, my water broke and my body began pushing. Wow, okay. (Luckily I'd been in the largest bathroom room that had handrails by the toilet, and tons of space with a chair in the corner – very nice bathroom, yes).

A few minutes later, our server knocked on the door (having been sent by my husband to check on me – and she told him, "I'll make sure she's not going into labor, ha ha"). I answered her between low pushing moans, saying, "would you please go get my husband?" Sensing the urgency, she rushed back to get Eric. He came in the room and saw that our baby was coming NOW, and he said, "Oh wow, okay." He had no time to panic, he was very ready, strong, and helpful. He saw baby's head coming out and reassured me that I was doing great, while I kept saying, "My baby. My baby."

Within just a few minutes, baby Christopher came out into the loving, surprised arms of his father. I threw my shirt onto the chair in the corner, and then held my baby against my bare chest to keep him warm. Our server came back with a tablecloth (for a blanket) and lots of towels.

I sat and held my baby for a while. Eric then called our Doula and told her our baby had come and asked if she would come meet us at the restaurant. She arrived and helped me clean up. Eric brought my stuff in from the car; the diapers, baby clothes, carseat, blanket, and everything I needed. We put the attached placenta in a Ziploc bag and wrapped it in a blanket with my baby. I was dressed and ready again and carried my baby back out into the restaurant. The owner of the restaurant and our serving team all gathered to take a picture with us.

We then went home to a very surprised babysitter, and showed our other two children their new baby brother. We celebrated and shared a chocolate cake, cut the cord, then went to sleep for the night with our precious new baby boy.

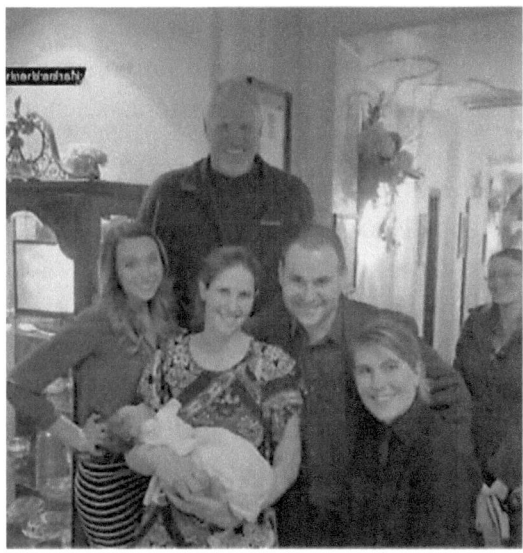

Picture taken with the overjoyed couple, the owner (back), the waitresses (far left and bottom right), and the Doula, the author of this book, Bree Moore (far right in the back).

Fast and Pleasurable
Submitted by Heather Bailey

DIANA
Born September 18th, 2017
Springville, Utah

Baby #1 and #2 were both born at local birth centers with midwives. #3 was a planned unassisted home birth with a surprise location, an Italian restaurant! (See Christopher's story: Birth Before Dinner)

This is Diana's story. Baby #4 comes with a simple story, yet exactly what I hoped for. For this birth, I considered hiring a midwife or Doula, yet in my heart of hearts I knew I wanted the birth to be simple and peaceful, with just me and my husband there together.

Since we had done this before, my husband was totally supportive. He, being a certified Hypnotherapist, even created a Hypnosis for me for a calm, peaceful, pleasurable birth. I wrote out my Ideal story, and he did a gentle hypnosis with me almost every night for the last few weeks before the birth.

I read many unassisted birth books, gathered all my baby and birthing supplies, and looked forward with hopeful anticipation.

September 13th, a beautiful fall day, started very normal with no strong signs of baby coming yet. Afternoon brought a few contractions. Later, as I finished washing dinner dishes, I started having to pause and breathe through the contractions as they came. I suspected my water had broken (not too sure), yet I was not totally convinced it was birthing time. I sat down with my family to watch a movie, and I had to continue closing my eyes, breathing through each contraction, rocking back and forth while leaning against the couch.

Right about 8 p.m., my 1-yr-old suddenly got super tired needed to go to bed immediately. I took him upstairs and laid him in his crib. After putting him to sleep, I realized I was not going back down to finish the movie. I asked my husband to come up, and he left the older two children to finish watching the movie. He arranged for my two younger brothers to watch our children in case they needed anything.

My husband and I went in our room. Eric filled our large tub with warm water, and I thought I'd be on the bed for a while, but all I wanted was to get into the warm water. Within 30 minutes, contractions intensified. I moaned, rocked back and forth, and tried to get comfortable in the water, but no position felt very good at all. One specific moment, I had the thought, "if I want to use the toilet before this birth, now is the last chance." I didn't want to have to move, so I just stayed in the tub, and within a few short minutes my body began pushing.

At this point, (as doubt always comes right before the reward), thoughts of doubt entered my mind, and I asked my husband, Eric, to keep telling me that I am amazing and capable, and that I could do this. He then readied himself, and gently reassured me as baby's head came out. The pushing intensified, intense, yet manageable, as long as it didn't last forever! My baby came, Eric reached in the water for her, then placed her in my arms. Calm and peace filled the room as I held my baby next to me in the warm water. I covered her with a small towel. We laid there in the water for almost an hour. Eric brought our Ashley and Bradley in to see their beautiful baby sister.

I birthed the placenta, and when I was ready, we wrapped baby Diana in a towel, I handed her to Eric, and he helped me out of the tub. I showered, then got dressed and held my baby again. We spent a little while longer together, then when I was ready, we all went to sleep for the night.

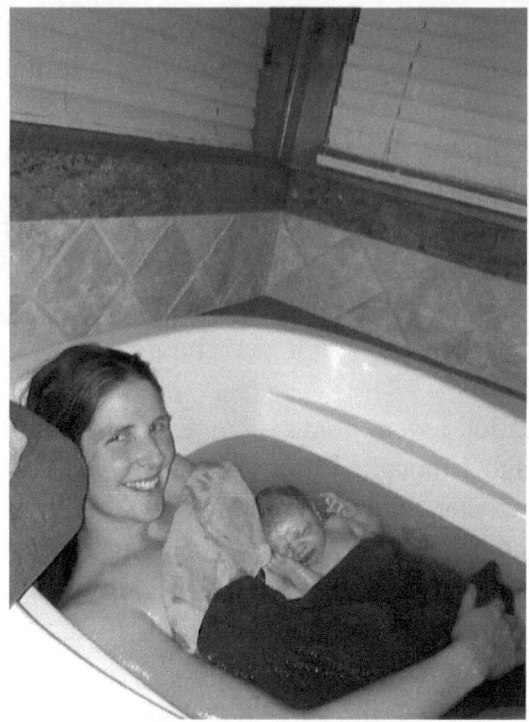

Heather and Diana

The Truth of the Wild Woman
Submitted by Marjorie S.

KENTUCKY

I was 20 when I gave birth to my first in a hospital with a CNM (certified nurse midwife). It was a longer-than-average labor (74 total hrs). At any other hospital I would've been sectioned. In the end I was punished. My baby was kidnapped by the NICU, and things happened to us without my consent. On the second day of our stay, I cried to my partner, "I'm never having another baby in the hospital." He agreed.

I got pregnant again in 2018. I provided my own medical care. I made my own decisions. Responsibility was totally in my hands. I was 22 when I gave birth to my second.

On November 27, 2018 at 9 a.m., my waters released slowly. My plug came and then my show. Slowly, waves started rolling in. I was smiling and happy, I nursed my oldest one final time, it's just the two of us. It's noon, we order a whole pizza and I eat it all. My mom comes around and I wax her face and my partner's eyebrows, there was lots of laughing and giggling.

Around 5 p.m. waves are becoming more regular, and I need to breath through them. The lights are off as I relax in between them. Around 7 p.m. transition starts hitting. I'm scared and beginning to doubt myself. The contractions are bringing on a high like no other. My partner provides support in his presence, but he keeps his hands away from me and gives me verbal encouragement, just what I need. The waves roll in as I begin to bear down with them.

I'm holding back because I'm scared of repeating what happened last time. My partner encourages me some more, and I know what I must do. I have to give in. I bear down with the waves, I can feel baby working with me. We do this for a while and my partner says he can see the baby. I stick a finger inside, and what I feel feels really soft. I have another contraction and suddenly need to be in the bathroom. I waddle in there with baby's head in my canal. I stand over the toilet and ask for a mirror. My partner brings it, and I look and I'm so so happy he was right, it was the head.

I start crying. I'm so ready to meet my baby. Seeing that sweet little head gave me the strength I needed. Any concern of being tired or laboring as long as last time melted away. I push and push. I scream and feel like a Wild Woman. Baby's head is born. I don't want to go on. Again my partner encourages me, another wave comes and his body flies out. My partner catches him over the toilet. The rest of my waters flow out with baby.

My partner passes him to me quickly. We are ecstatic. I look at my baby, such a beautiful face. There is nothing like the eyes of a fresh newborn. My baby gazes back at me and gurgles. We both sigh relief and laugh. Instinctively, I suction him with my mouth. He coughs and clears more from his lungs. Every single cell in my body surges with joy, life and love. Baby has great color as I rub the vernix in.

Finally, I look and yell out to my partner (he was tending the toddler) that we had another boy. This moment made my life. About 5 or 10 minutes after birth, and I have a gush of blood. I know this is my placenta. Contractions come back and I push with one. The placenta comes out with more blood and fluids. It felt so heavy and an incredible pleasure to release. Finally, I get to rest in bed and nurse my new baby. I can't stop smiling. I'm on such a high. I gave birth finally, it didn't happen to me, it wasn't done to me. I got to experience the Truth. The truth of my body, the truth of the wisdom of the earth.

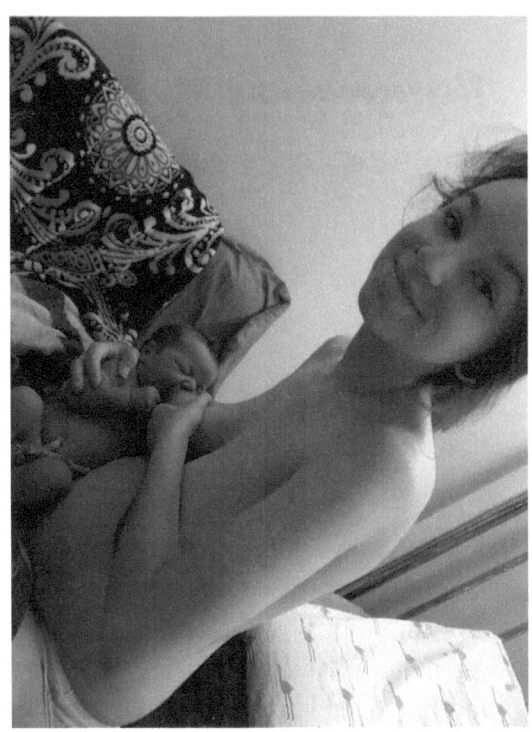

Reprogramming My Brain
Submitted by Annalise Jones

MY FIRST BIRTH WAS in 2005, a managed home birth. I didn't have any expectations other than staying out of the hospital. I thought I was taking care of my health and well-prepared since I had followed all my prenatal advice and even read a few books about natural birthing and practiced some things. But looking back, I was so young and naïve. My biggest mistake was failing to prepare myself spiritually to own my own birth experience.

Honestly, it didn't occur to me. It's sad that in our society, moms hire birth assistants and then become pretty passive. Even if I had a birth plan and felt in control of important decisions, I was very passive psychologically in that I was giving over the power of this birth and depending on somebody else. Then again, what can first time moms realistically do? I was only 21 years old. You learn from experience.

That first birth was a "successful" yet fairly traumatic home birth, as I hemorrhaged and went into shock, and had the baby taken from me for respiratory treatment. As a result of this busy-ness and my anxiety, I didn't bond with my baby for an hour afterward. I was so consumed with my own complications that it didn't occur to me to hold or nurse my baby. I called my mom on the phone and she had to tell me to do so. I was pretty disconnected, out of the fear of having to transfer to the hospital.

In 2007 I found an amazing blog written by a hands-off midwife and learned about natural physiology and protecting the bubble in the 3rd stage of labor. I poured over this blog, completely thrilled with what I was reading. It made so much sense! I was able to identify what went wrong with my mismanaged birth. I felt betrayed by a midwife who was supposed to support me and promote healthy outcomes but instead caused my complications. I regretted deeply that I hadn't been able to hold and bond with my baby immediately after birth, and that my midwife was uneducated about natural placenta birth.

At the same time in my life, I was learning about nutrition – REAL nutrition, not just getting a certain amount of protein each day, drinking herbal tea and calling it good. I got myself healthy. I lost 65 pounds and felt radiant, younger, and healthier than ever. I was amazed at the healing capabilities of our bodies and I knew my body was perfectly able to do what it was made to do – build and bring forth healthy babies!

That year we moved to a new city and I got pregnant again. I had been in touch with multiple midwives who agreed with the hands-off philosophy. My prenatal care consisted of lots of emails asking questions, eating superbly well to ensure I was energetic and feeling positive, and doing lots of emotional healing work. Essentially, I had to reprogram my brain with a new belief system that birth was quick, easy, painless and straightforward. Because of these things, I was in an ideal spiritual place, filled with faith in creation and my body. I was very confident that the birth would go well.

I was planning an unassisted birth, but ready to call my midwife friends if we had questions. One of them was able to lend me some equipment so I was thankful for this safety net. One thing I spent a lot of time on was researching hemorrhage and preparing for the possibility of it happening again. I basically taught myself all the things I wish that first midwife would have known, like how to birth the placenta quickly to minimize bleeding. I also took some herbs to build my blood and various other supplements I needed for my overall health and hormone balance. I was also very prepared to deal with infant respiratory issues.

I went into labor the very day of my due date. I was swinging my toddler son at the park when I felt the first contraction. It was late morning. My mom was with us so it worked out perfectly. We went back to the house and I busied myself preparing lunch and snacks to last the rest of the day, then went upstairs and set up the birthing area. Contractions were progressing steadily so I went ahead with my birth plan. I texted my husband to finish up his work, and put on Josh Groban to sing and dance to. Dancing in labor is the best! Swaying the hips really helps, and psychologically I became mesmerized with my own body. My husband came home around 1:00 p.m. and I quickly explained the various items I had lying around. We got the bathtub filled and were sensual with each other during contractions.

Since my first birth had been a water birth, I was curious to try a land birth. But when I got out of the tub on my hands and knees for a contraction, I quickly changed my mind! The warm water felt sooooo nice. I had made a deal with myself to think positive and not say a single negative thing. I had spent a lot of my first labor whining, feeling unsure. But this approach was completely different. I was filled with faith, hope, and excitement. I talked to my baby as we worked together, saying encouraging things as teammates would in a sporting event. My husband was a great support, giving me what I needed and keeping cool washcloths on my shoulders. But it really didn't last long. I had programmed myself for a fast, easy birth and that's exactly what I got.

At one point I felt inside myself and felt the head. It was such an incredible rush! I was taking care of myself and yet surrendering to the process of nature. Such a beautiful paradox of self-reliance. I wanted my son to witness the birth so I told my husband to go get him, but then another contraction came and I said, "No! Don't leave!" It was only a few pushes before the baby launched out all at once like a rocket. I caught her myself (I was kneeling/squatting) and knew exactly what to do. I held her over my arm and rubbed her back to get her breathing. After a minute she pinked up and looked terrific. She never cried.

I yelled downstairs that the baby was born! Come see! My mother was very surprised because she hadn't heard anything, and it had only been a couple hours since I first went upstairs to prepare. It was a very special time for my mother and me to share this experience. The pinnacle of womanhood. She told me I was her hero.

I continued holding my baby as my husband cut a bite of placenta for me to eat, and internally I spoke with my placenta and released it. Once it was birthed, I got up and carried her to the bed and sat up against pillows to get her nursing. We nursed for an hour while talking, snacking, and making phone calls. I cannot describe the high I felt. I got the exact birth I wanted (I had visualized and programmed my mind for this) and it was an incredible triumph to have a completely natural physiological birth with no hold ups, no complications, and she never left my arms for the first few hours of life. She was my precious jewel.

Calling my dad was funny. He was a little taken back that there was no midwife. He said, "So, your husband delivered her?" and I retorted, "No way! I delivered her!" Nobody was going to take my power from me. Funny how we are all conditioned to believe that somebody has to "deliver" the baby. If only we could understand once and for all, that babies come out. They have been doing so for thousands of years. Nobody knows better than my own body. How many women are missing out on the joy and empowerment of owning their own birth experience? It's weird to think, even my best friends have no idea what they're missing out on.

A couple hours after the birth we got around to cutting the cord, weighing her, and calling my in-laws who lived locally. They remarked how fresh I looked, like I hadn't just given birth. I felt incredibly healthy and vibrant. As I write this, that day was over 7 years ago, and it remains the most wonderful day of my life.

Quick and Intense
Submitted by Annalise Jones

A FEW YEARS LATER, I was pregnant for the third time. I was in a slightly different place in life—still eating very well, but also working out heavily, running a full time business out of my home, and homeschooling my two older kids. I was one busy lady! I didn't have time for much journaling or visualizing, and didn't feel in touch with my spiritual side the same way as before. But I figured UC *(unassisted childbirth)* was old hat, and we would just have this baby. Somehow I knew the baby would come early. We bought my mom's flights but I told her she wouldn't make it. The due date was January 7. We got Christmas done with and mentally moved on to the next event: Let's get this baby born!

The night of December 28th, I started some prodromal labor and kept resting/snoozing, and I timed contractions. They weren't really going anywhere. So I slept. The next day I had some work to finish up with my business. I spent all morning unpacking cases of merchandise, and getting things squared away to take a few days off. Contractions puttered on. It's like they were waiting for me to be ready.

Sure enough, as soon as the house was cleaned up after lunch, active labor began. Contractions were suddenly every 3 minutes. We called a midwife friend whom I wanted to help with the birth, and brought the kids over to my in-law's house. When the midwife showed up my contractions really slowed down. I walked down the street and back. I admit I was aware of the show I was putting on (with my facial expressions, etc. as she watched). We visited for a half hour or so and my labor seemed to have stopped. Well, I felt embarrassed! I laid down in bed and rested for a while, and we told her she could leave. Well, what do you know, as soon as we did that, labor began again in earnest! It's funny, I thought labor had stopped so I was calling my sister for a chat. I was pretty relaxed, and she was getting into a story when I felt some hard contractions and I kind of panicked. I had to end that phone call but I'm not one to be rude!

I told her suddenly, "Sorry, but I gotta go!" And thus began an hour of very intense labor. Contractions were hard and came on very strong, one after the next. I was standing up, arms around my husband's shoulders, rocking and moaning. This labor was not calm and gentle like my last! It was very intense.

I got into the bath tub. Exhausted, I panted in between contractions. I was crying out to God, feeling like I was about to be ripped in half. Soon enough I had a pushing urge and after a few pushes, he shot out like a rocket (same as my last birth) sunny-side up! I remember watching his face emerge. He cried loud right away for a few minutes. I was so exhausted, I just held him in my arms and took some breaths. I couldn't put him to the breast right away because he was crying. My mother-in-law came over right away with the older kids and saw me in all my glory, naked in a bloody bath with floating poop. That's a memory I'm proud of. Haha!

Unbeknownst to me, my husband had texted the midwife and asked her to come back. She let herself in right after the birth and said hello, then sat in the other room and knitted until we asked for her. My mother-in-law was suspicious and wondered why she wasn't doing anything (we hadn't ever told my in-laws about UC). It must have been a pretty interesting scene from the perspective of somebody used to a busy medical birth. Here I was just chilling out with my baby in a nasty bath while the "care provider" (as she saw her) knitted in the other room!

When my mother-in-law asked what was going on, I said we were waiting for the placenta. She said "Well, shouldn't she be doing something to get it out?" Haha. Anyway she left, and then I got up and delivered the placenta on the toilet. We went to bed and my midwife friend cleaned up, weighed him, cut the cord, etc. and we nursed. (I definitely recommend having somebody to clean up and help with all that business! The first UC it was my mom and we didn't spend a dime. But this second time we paid my friend for her help). My husband cooked. It was dinnertime, and I was starving!

In hindsight, looking at the intensity and exhaustion of this labor, my body was not fresh for childbirth after being so busy-busy-busy. Now I know to take more rest and time to care for myself leading up to birth. I also know that my body does NOT like anybody besides my husband around, and I won't bother trying that again.

A note about my children's personalities: they all match their birth. My first born has had some emotional imbalances and we've done a lot of healing work. My daughter, the first UC, is a calm, sensitive introvert. My other son, the second UC, is very busy-body, active and intense.

Beautiful Harmony and Sweet Surrender
Submitted by Annalise Jones

FRIDAY I HAD A moving conversation with someone and felt that this baby was ready but might need a jump start. I had mixed feelings as I usually over-analyze everything, so I went to pray. I asked the Lord if I should take the homeopathic pills I had been considering all week—if so I need a sign. Could you give me a contraction now?

Right away I felt a BH (Braxton Hicks) tightening. So I took the pills and noted the time—I would need to take a dose every 20 mins for a couple hours. I also looked up some YouTube videos and while watching a movie held various acupressure points. By the end of the movie I recognized some true (not BH) contractions. I lay down to go to bed and felt a series of them. I fell asleep open to the possibility of waking up to labor. But I guess I needed to keep up with the pills maybe. I slept pretty well, feeling some throughout the night. But by 6 a.m. I felt confident sending my partner, Rychen, out on his 3-hour marathon training run.

I had this prodromal labor all morning. Really irregular contractions. I didn't take the pills again yet because I wanted to make a spicy curry lunch, which might antidote them. We were busy with a few things anyway. So early afternoon I took homeopathics again. It gave me a push but there was still no regular pattern. I found it significant that between 3:30-4:30 while I lay on the couch I timed consistent contractions about 5 minutes apart. But as soon as I got up and moved they went back to being off/on, irregular both in frequency, duration and intensity.

Rychen and I lay down to watch a TV show and they really fizzled out it seemed. Plus I was getting sleepy and not in the mood for games!

Ate dinner, discussed false labor with my mom who had 8 kids and had her fair share. I thought that's what it was and felt pretty down. Just wanted to go to bed and try tomorrow. I had to give Elisabeth a shower first and I had a few successive contractions there.

After giving her a shower I got in the bath per mom's advice to try to make the "false labor" stop. I just felt down so I called my cousin Alyssa for a pep talk since she is a birth warrior with six kids! Contractions did not stop.

Couldn't decide if I wanted to walk and encourage it or just rest. I guess a part of me wasn't ready for it to get going and I still felt tired and a bit despondent, so I rested in bed. Felt a strong contraction in my hips and was like "Back labor? No thank you!" So I crawled on my hands and knees up and down the hallway to flip the baby, all while giving the two older kids instructions for going to bed. They needed so much attention and I was getting irritable! Just go to bed and let me deal with labor! (My 10-year-old said "you're not in labor"—I guess he expected me to be louder?)

After putting them to bed I just wanted to lay and snooze and hopefully get through the night, since it still didn't seem like serious labor. My husband and I lay down (about 8:30 p.m.) and I had a few strong contractions, enough to hold his hand and really focus on my breathing. In my mind I said "I surrender. I allow myself to open and my baby to come down."

I guess that psychological conceding was just the trick I needed because right away things really picked up and I felt a lot of pressure. I thought I must have to go the bathroom, and while I was standing in the bathroom I was overcome by a series of intense contractions. I just stood in the bathroom hanging on to my husband! My sucking urge kicked in and I sucked his hand a bit (is that just me? I get this oral fixation in labor) I must have been in transition. Which means all the irregularity was in fact "active labor."

We filled the tub and I got in. We let our birth team know things were for real. These intense contractions continued one on top of the other for about an hour. I gnawed on my husbands thumb with each one!

When he needed to grab something there'd be a little hesitation as I clung to him, and I'd tell him when I was ready for him to jump up quick. But it's interesting when communication is difficult! For example I was getting cold but couldn't express that. I turned on the hot water myself—the bath was already full but it felt nice to have a hot stream I could touch. Another time I wanted a stimulating oil and reached to my selection to find peppermint (honestly for some reason it's easier to attempt doing the action myself than to say the words "peppermint oil"!) but I managed to communicate it and he began giving me whiffs of peppermint and lemon for mental vigor. He also put a small pillow on the bath ledge which was nice to put my forehead on.

As we neared pushing, my body naturally began panting and shaking with the contractions. I could feel the head about 2 inches inside me, with a large cervical lip. So for about 20 minutes, I focused hard with each contraction, visualizing the lip going back and praying, and saying "I release this, I release any and all blocks or hesitancy that could be involved," etc.

I kept checking myself every few contractions, but I had mixed feelings because it would bring on a stronger one each time afterward. So, finally, I felt the lip gone and got a good feel of the head—hair and some kind of a funny ridge. I thought baby might not be presenting ideally. So I focused with each contraction on talking to baby. "Chin down please!" And in between I stood up to move my hips around, such as putting one foot up on the bath ledge in a deep side lunge position. Then as each contraction began I would kneel back down in the water and pant some more and grasp my husband.

It's interesting how people say "try to let your body push by itself, go slowly, just pant," and I was keeping that in mind, although I wasn't really controlling what I was doing. My body automatically did the panting, and I didn't have a strong pushing urge. I think only twice (not consecutively) did I feel the need to give a push, and they are big pushes with a loud roar!! Of course this meant clearing my bowels the first one which actually felt nice to relieve some pressure.

I felt a stretch as the head emerged, and then my body stopped for a minute and just rested. It was a new experience for me—my other two unhindered births, they were smaller and just shot out all at once like rockets! So I thought it was funny to have a head out, just chilling! (I considered standing up out of the water to show Rychen. Good thing I didn't because in retrospect, I remember the fact that the baby would have taken its first breath and it would be dangerous to get back down in the water.)

So after a minute another contraction came and the rest slid out. Always an amazing, indescribable moment! All I could do was shout, "oh my gosh, oh my gosh!" And lift baby up. I held baby across my arm, face down. It was 10:00 p.m. Baby snorted her first breath and then got real quiet and I realized she had slept through her birth! She lay contentedly in my arms for several minutes as we called in everyone to come see (including my friend who lives close by who wanted to come as soon as possible!). After my friend arrived we all peeked together and saw it was a girl!!

I got out for the placenta to be delivered, walked around, but since the bleeding was fine I thought why hurry? I need to lay down and rest. But after a few minutes I changed my mind. I know people who wait and let it come leisurely, but I'd just rather have it over with! So I followed Lennon's tips, and it took longer than previous times but it finally came out about 10:45. All the while holding (nursing some) baby attached to me. I wasn't opposed to cutting the cord but it just didn't happen with the various hubbub.

Again, I had to talk to myself and release any subconscious beliefs blocking it.They say letting the placenta go is the final goodbye to pregnancy and sometimes we resist that. Could have been true for me, this pregnancy was a long road with lots of learning, growth, and faith. The last couple weeks really weren't bad at all. It was like a friendship I had come to appreciate.

Finally, I got to lay down and nurse my baby. Lennon took care of the cord, helping my 10-year old to cut it. I had some snacks and Lennon finished things up (cleaning, giving me advice, etc) and a while later weighed baby at 8 lbs 14 oz (I delayed taking the baby from me because she would cry out loudly when she was disturbed) and we put the kids to bed (again!) at now 1:00 a.m.

My husband went down to eat his dinner while I just marveled at the whole thing!! Birth is so amazing. Our bodies are created in such beautiful harmonies, and it's a wonderful thing to experience pure, undisturbed instinct. To be the one "in charge" of my own birth and yet surrender because I am really just a passenger as God works his glory through me. Childbirth is truly the pinnacle of a woman's creation. It's such an honor to experience it.

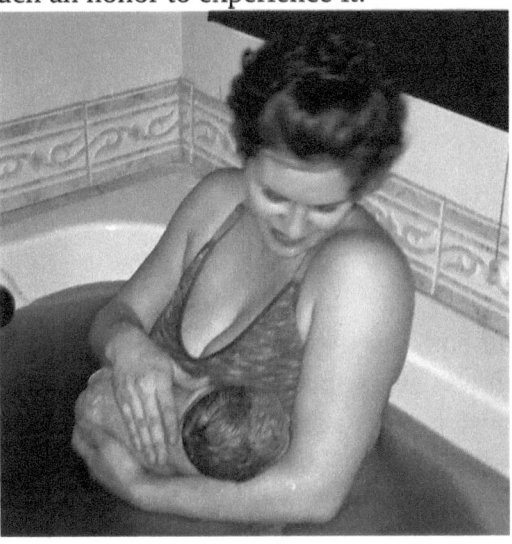

Fast, Pleasurable Birth of Odena
Submitted by Robye Albrecht

ODENA SAYLOR
May 24th, 2018

The time had come to try for one more baby, and I had plans to ensure my birth was everything I didn't get with my past births. Like many who choose to go unassisted, I had a bad experience the time before with doctors taking over my birth plan. This time around I would have my midwife during the prenatal care, but I would birth without her or any other medical professionals involved.

The day was like any other, relaxing and watching television. I had my pool blown up and my supply basket ready, candles out and the hose hooked to the shower. I did all of this three weeks early. At 38 weeks 5 days I was talking on the phone to my mom and all of a sudden my water broke! I was so excited and told her to hurry up because I have precipitous (fast) labors. My mother was two hours away, and my grandma was visiting. My boyfriend was three hours away at work, so I called him right away.

My two daughters were home with me. It was 7:06 p.m. I called my 11-year-old into the room as I was on the toilet. I told her my water broke and to help me set up. I laid some blankets down in the living room and put the pool on top and then had my daughter start filling it up. I headed to the bathroom to do my hair and makeup. A few of my friends wanted to come and experience this with me, and so I started calling them and then had my daughter take over while I finished getting ready.

One friend, Christina, showed up and was so nervous, but she did an awesome job following directions and helping my daughter prepare. I set up my iPad for Facebook Live so all my family could watch, and by this time contractions had started. They were like period pains and not strong at all, but I got in my pool anyway. My other friend, Krissy, called and was trying to get over quickly. She had been to both of my other births. She asked my friend if I was screaming and in a lot of pain. Christina said, "No, she is meditating in the pool with her headphones on." So, naturally Krissy assumed she had time!

Well, she showed up very shortly, and by now I had my 3-year-old swimming with me in the pool and contractions were around two minutes apart, but still not painful. My boyfriend is watching on Facebook and on his way home. My mom is also watching and driving down, and my sister is eating snacks and watching my live feed.

Krissy arrives, and I ask for more hot water. As she is filling up more hot water, my friend Ashley arrives. All these friends and still no mom or boyfriend!

Let me add, I never once had any fear or anxiety or negative thoughts. I was full of excitement and empowering feelings and trust in myself.

Well, I have the urge to go number two, and I would have never assumed it was close to pushing time because everything was still so pain free. I get up to go to the toilet and after going my body pushes. I feel a big bulge, and she is in position! I yell, "I am crowning!" and my daughter was so funny. When I looked back at the video, she is jumping up and down saying mom is going to have her in the toilet! They yell at me to get back in the pool; well I need help walking, ha ha. I get in and Ashley is still shocked since we just called her about an hour ago!

I still have my meditation music on with my Bluetooth headphones, and I am back in the pool with my body pushing on its own. I reach down, and she is crowning. I ask where Luke is at and say, "It's not time baby, just wait, it's not time." I allow my body to do short slow pushing and all this time I can't even feel a contraction, only pushing. I am telling her to go slow so I don't tear.

I hear my friends say, "What should we do? Should we grab her?"
I shout, "Don't touch her!" without any control.
They say, "You got this mama."
Finally her head is out! I will never forget my 3-year-old say, "My sister, it's my sister." So much oxytocin came over me and with one last push she was out. I brought her up onto my chest. Out of instinct I sucked some stuff from her mouth, and she let out a cry. My friends grabbed the towels from the dryer and then Demetra, my friend, came walking in. Everyone shouts you would miss this! Ha ha, she is always late to things. She asked how I was feeling and my response was, "I am great!"

Ondena Saylor was born at 8:14 p.m.

I moved to the bed to deliver my placenta, and that sucker took just as long as my entire labor to get out. During that time, my mom, grandma, and boyfriend showed up and they were so proud and said they watched it (live) and couldn't wait to get to the house. My friend Demetra helped with all the placenta stuff. We finally cut the cord after delivering the placenta (1 hour 20 minutes).

This was the most amazing experience; my fastest birth yet, and it was pain free! If it could be like this every time I would keep having babies!

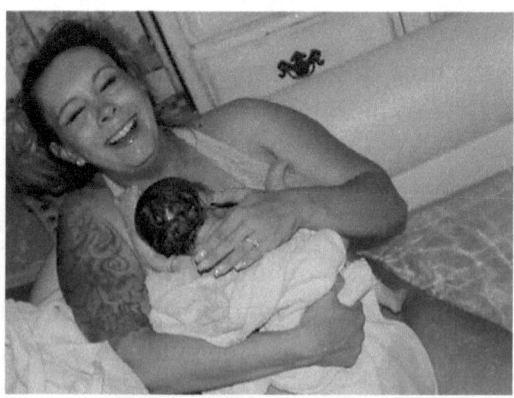

First-time Birth, First-time Freebirth
Submitted by Tatiana Derichsweiler

OREGON, USA

I closed my eyes and leaned back against the tub. I was tired, rightfully so. But I was also utterly, blissfully, relaxed and delighted. I could feel his little body squirm as I held his naked body against mine. I could feel the oxytocin coursing through my body, creating a "birth high." It was a deep soul satisfying feeling. If I'm being honest, that feeling lasted for months…

Let's back up a little. I'm a first time mother that chose a freebirth. Not very common. Sometime in the night between Sunday and Monday I started having contractions. By 4 a.m. I couldn't sleep. Around 5 a.m. I started timing them. They were lasting about a minute but were eight minutes apart. By 8 a.m. They were only 45 seconds long but seven minutes apart. I lounged in bed that morning and ate a big breakfast.

I went to the store and picked up all the little last minute things we might need and ran some errands. I went to an acupuncture appointment from 11-12:30 and walked home from there. I finished setting up the birthing room and then worked in the garden doing the last of the planting then sat on the porch enjoying the cool night. We had dinner, and I tried to rest some so I would have energy for later.

By 10 p.m. the contractions were starting to pick up in intensity. They had been 4-5 minutes apart for hours at that point. I labored in the shower around midnight with contractions 2-3 minutes apart. I got in bed again after and tried to rest some. Around 2 a.m., I got up and did circuits between the living room and kitchen as the contractions kicked up another level.

I hit transition around 3 a.m. and threw up in the kitchen sink. I had been snacking all night to keep up energy levels, so I had a lot to bring up. I asked my other half to set up the tub, as I now started to vocalize through contractions. He started putting up the tub at 3:30 a.m. at my request, but we ran out of warm water at about five inches deep. I went to the bathroom at 3:45 a.m. and FER kicked in. Pop! The bag of waters burst and life water flowed down my legs.

I walked to the pool as soon as it was ready around 4 a.m. Once I lowered myself in, baby was already almost out. I called my partner over to take part in delivering our son. Only a few pushes in the pool, and the head was out. There was nuchal cord around his neck, but we couldn't unwrap it until his body was out.

We waited for my body to push out the rest of baby and realized as he came out that he had wrapped his leg and foot in the cord as well. We unraveled it all and passed him through my legs for me to pick him up. We sat back and relaxed. He had tons of vernix on his back. When I was ready, we birthed the placenta and relaxed some more. We got out of the tub and got into bed. I had one small graze (tear) that didn't need anything. Only 7 lbs 10 oz, 20.5in long, born Tuesday at 4:11 a.m. after less than 30 minutes of total pushing. We settled in for the night. Baby latched immediately upon seeing nipple and is a champion nurser. He's super alert and interactive for a newborn.

Birth can be unpredictable; but it's also raw, it's fierce, it's beautiful, and it's so incredibly empowering. My labor and delivery was the most empowering and magical experience of my life.

The Painless Birth of Alexis Will
Submitted by Carla Moyer

ALEXIS WILL
July 2012

When I got pregnant with my first baby, I was renting a room in a huge shared house with some 14 housemates. Mostly people kept to themselves, and most people thought my plans for freebirth were none of their business. Two of them cornered us in the kitchen before the birth to tell us that we couldn't do it, that the pain would be too much for me, that Dustin, my partner and another housemate would panic and faint, blah blah blah. It was annoying, but their ridiculous bug-eyed expressions and preposterous suggestions made me feel generally more confident about my decision.

I felt great for the entire pregnancy and was able to go out and do things until the very end. One of my housemates was moving out and his car broke down, and I was able to fix it for him (a very simple repair) when I was 9 months pregnant! I could still run (slower) and climb and jump around, so I felt confident the pregnancy was going very well. I did not want an ultrasound because it was just unnecessary exposure to powerful soundwaves, and would not cause me to make any decisions differently. Prenatal care did not seem necessary because I felt perfectly fine (but crabby), and checked my blood pressure at the drugstore, and it was always fine.

At the end of the pregnancy, I could feel a round hard head through the wall of my vagina, so I knew the baby was head down. Intuitively, I felt completely happy and calm with my decision, and if

I ever imagined going to the hospital instead, my chest would start to tighten and my breathing would get shallow.

I went into labor at 40 weeks and 6 days. Those six days were terribly long and frustrating. I was tired of being pregnant and uncomfortable and wanted to see my baby. Finally, as I was getting in bed at around midnight, I had little a contraction that felt like light menstrual cramps and a tightening in my belly. Five minutes later I had another, and five minutes after that, another. I said to Dustin that I thought it was finally starting, and he smiled and looked encouraging. The lights were low and soft and he timed the contractions for the first few hours; they were almost exactly six minutes apart, and lasted a minute, and would stay at that spacing and duration for the next 23 hours until delivery.

The first twelve hours of labor, until about noon the next day (July 23, 2012) were very easy. I mostly laid in bed and would rock from side to side with my legs. The contractions were almost completely painless as long as I kept moving. By about noon, the contractions had begun to ramp up in intensity, and I found I actually had to get up and sway my weight from one foot to the other to keep them from hurting. At this point, I had never wanted to go to sleep more in my entire life. All I could think about was how tired I was and that I could tell I wasn't even close to delivering. I knew there were many hours to go before I'd be done, so between contractions I would lie down like I was dead to conserve my energy.

Once, I tried to stay laying down in hospital position instead of getting up and swaying like I had been. The pain was like hellfire daggers and drove me to my feet in a second. Once swaying, the pain was down to almost nothing again. It was incredible! I didn't really make noise because the contractions weren't particularly painful, so none of my housemates knew what was up.

For the duration of my labor, Dustin sat in the corner of the room and was apparently terrified but didn't show it. At one point, I asked him to drag our mattress into a darker part of the room and to cover the windows with sheets so it wouldn't be so bright.

At about 6 p.m., 18 hours from the initial contraction, they really started to get intense. I was still tired, and still mad that I hadn't gotten any sleep, and still trying to conserve every calorie of energy I had. I really had to thrash around pretty violently to keep the contractions from hurting, and sometimes they even got the best of me and the pain would spike in about the 6/10 range for bursts of 20 seconds at a time. I found it was best to be on my big wide mattress so I could roll and thrash, and rest comfortably in between during this period.

At about 8 p.m. the sun started to get low in the sky. I went for a pee break and on the toilet when I wiped, I felt what felt like a water balloon bulging out of my vagina. "Oh good, things are getting close." I relayed the info to Dustin when I got back to our room, and he was happy to hear it. I had been having contractions perfectly spaced every five to six minutes, consistently ramping up in intensity but never feeling the urge to push. I started to wonder when I was supposed to, but I didn't have a lot of mental energy to think about it. Then, one contraction to the next, my body was suddenly pushing as hard as it could. It doubled me over with the force of it. "This must be the part where I push." I just went with it, helping as much as I felt like with my conscious effort.

The sac didn't last long with the pushing, and when it popped, only a little fluid came out. Her head must have been right at the bottom of my birth canal holding all the waters back behind her. The pushing contractions were not particularly painful, and I lay and rocked a little through them. The sound I made was involuntary straining, like a cartoon character pushing an impossibly heavy weight. I still felt perfectly, completely good and nearly pain free, but still begrudging the no sleep.

Eventually, it got completely dark and I remember being surprised and a little bit worried about how long it was lasting. I wondered how much longer it might be. At this point I was sitting in a recliner, still pushing and wondering if it was ever going to get finished with, and I'd get to finally go to sleep. I was slouched back with my knees bent and my feet on the seat of the chair. I saw my vulva bulge. With the next contraction and push, the bulge came out a little farther. Absolutely no pain. A couple of contractions in, and all I could see of the bulge was my own flesh. I had a sudden hysterically irrational thought that the baby was not lined up with my cervix and could tear through my tissues…with absolutely no pain, right? Dustin was crouched on the floor watching at this point and I babbled this to him, and he said "I see hair!" so I told him to take a picture and show me. He did and all fear disappeared, and I was back to business.

After a handful of pushes, the head was bulging most of the way out, and I had the sudden urge to get up. I told Dustin to move, and I hopped up with surprisingly little effort and stood in a gentle squat for the next push. The head emerged and I actually felt like I was clenching down on her to hold her in. I asked Dustin if he wanted to catch the baby, and he put his hand about an inch away from the head to catch. I couldn't explain in time what I meant, and it felt like the baby was going to fall out on the floor, so I pushed his hand away and put the flat of my hand on the head and held it back in place, waiting for the next contraction.

The last push delivered her all at once, and I had to hold her back so she didn't come out too fast. I was hunched over and saw her body twist as it was pushed through my pelvis. When her first arm was freed, it dropped suddenly towards the floor, which triggered her startle reflex and made her make a surprised squawk. She was facing away from me at the time, and so before I even saw her face I knew she was alive and well. On her arm I thought I saw a tiny blob of blood. She was a lovely pink and otherwise completely clean, and not even particularly slippery. I allowed the hand that was on her head to slide down to her upper chest, and I caught the rest of her with my other hand. I held her against my chest, leaned my head on the mattress on the floor in front of me and caught my breath, and in that moment Dustin snapped a fantastic picture.

When I stood up, I was holding a lovely, perfect, six pound little girl. It did not hurt the slightest bit, and she was looking at me with bright little eyes. I saw the blob of blood on her arm was actually a birthmark that she shares with her great grandmother. Same shape, same spot. Dustin was standing right next to me and a second after standing, all the amniotic waters gushed out of me mixed with the delivery blood. We looked at each other with wide eyes, but I was fine - it was mostly water and very little blood from the look of it. It would look worse to someone who doesn't have periods.

I toweled off and sat down and just held my new, beautiful Alexis. Not long after, Dustin had stepped out to get the bathroom ready for us, and I felt the placenta coming. I got up out of my chair holding the baby in one arm, squatted, and delivered the placenta into my other hand. It felt soft and hot. Squatted over, everything felt very safe and balanced held against my chest. But I did not feel safe standing up. I looked across the the long chasm of my room at the placenta bowl on my dresser and laughed. "Dustin! Could you come back?"

Some time after, Dustin had left again to finish getting the bath ready and I heard a tiny knock on my door. It was my landlady, Julia, who had been out on the back porch, and close enough to my open window to hear me pushing and a few baby sounds. She was from Zimbabwe and had six children, including one unassisted that happened faster than she could react, so she was all smiles and congratulations. Some 45 minutes after the baby was born, my fool housemate, the same one who freaked out at me in the kitchen, calls an emergency nurse! The nurse freaks out and is trying to send us an ambulance, and Dustin is irritated and trying to calm her down and reassure her that we do not need help and that the baby looks excellent.

Eventually our end of the house is a quiet buzz, and I walk naked, holding my baby, with blood streaked down my legs to the bathroom. Dustin follows close behind holding the placenta, still attached to Alexis. About four completely awestruck housemates follow gingerly behind, whispering if it's okay for them to come in to see the baby. I say yes, and the few folks that are up come in one by one for a few minutes and are generally amazed. None of them heard a thing and had no idea the labor was happening.

We washed off in the bath, and Alexis made a tiny sneeze that made everyone in the room whisper-squeal. After a little while, she made her first little cry, so I put her to my breast. She pulled my whole nipple in her mouth and sucked in little flutters. It was a strange feeling, ever so slightly unpleasant but mostly fine. She nursed for a nice long stretch, and eventually, I felt tired of being in the water and also tired of having a placenta on the baby.

It had been about an hour and a half at that point, and we tied the strings we'd prepared around the cord and cut in the middle. The cord was completely white and had the tiniest red dot in the middle, and the placenta was cold and seemed extremely "finished" with it's job. She hardly cried at all, and even spent the occasional awake moment not nursing and just looking around the room with her bright little eyes.

Freebirthing Twins

"Love is unselfishly choosing for another's highest good."
- *C.S. Lewis*

The Births of Tristan Karl and Weston Troy
Submitted by Carla Moyer

IT WAS ONE DAY into the 38th week, a Tuesday, and contractions finally started that late afternoon. I had never been more hyperextended in my life. I hadn't slept well for weeks, and I could hardly eat or drink anything but the raw cow milk we were buying from a neighbor. I had spent all day, every day in an easy chair for the last two months of this pregnancy, with my only goals being to survive and bring my babies as close to term as I could take them. I couldn't stand for more than five minutes without all the ligaments in my lower belly screaming for me to sit down again. I couldn't even sit comfortably; sitting pushed my uterus up into my ribs so hard it felt like I was being cut.

Contractions were extremely gentle and never settled into a regular pattern. I tried standing up and swaying to ease the pain like with my singleton labor. But, I was so heavy and in so much pain that I couldn't, even if I hadn't been in labor. So I sat in my easy chair, and tried to sway side to side the best I could. It was unpleasant, but not measurably different than the misery of the last two months.

Contractions progressed erratically for about seven hours until midnight, and then stopped. I was happy for the chance to get a night's sleep. I only managed a few hours, being so horrendously full of squirming babies. Wednesday morning began, as usual, sipping coffee in my easy chair. By 10:00 a.m. contractions resumed, and I actually started to feel a little smug: the schedule was so leisurely and convenient!

Well, the contractions never settled into a pattern. Sometimes one would start to feel a little strong, but usually they were weak. Sometimes the spacing started to get close but then they'd drift apart again. I switched from my chair to my bed, never comfortable, never finding a movement or position where I could be at ease.

24 hours later, 10:00 a.m. Thursday, my husband came in to keep me company. I did not feel any closer to delivery, and had no idea if this was even true labor. I didn't feel trance like, and nothing was intensifying. I was not interested in doing cervical checks because I did not want to contaminate my vagina. I spent that morning and afternoon the same way: moving between my bed and chair, trying and failing to get comfortable, but at least having a sympathetic ear to complain to.

At 4:45 p.m., I felt like the clouds were parting; almost like I was coming back OUT of labor. I started to feel a creeping sense of hopelessness, like this was a purgatory I would never be free from. I stood for one last contraction, and tried to sit when it ended, but it was uncomfortable like I was sitting on something. So I stood back up and felt myself; my heart leapt, the bag was bulging!

From this point, I'd had only a few hours to go with my single, and I said to my husband that we were probably going to be at the finish line soon! Then I tried the tiniest push, like passing an almost imperceptible fart. The sac bulge suddenly became a crowning that filled my entire hand, and before I could even say to start videoing, the baby was expelled, sac and all!

I felt an instant urgency to burst the sac, even though it was seriously the coolest thing I'd ever seen, and I wanted to take pictures so badly. It was a glowing translucent yellow, and covered with tiny veins - prehistoric comes to mind. I didn't have free hands, so I told my husband to burst it, which he did immediately.

He said that as he was fumbling for a pinch hold on the membrane, that he saw the baby's screaming face float to the edge. He could hear him even though he was yelling in amniotic fluid and not air! As the sac burst, I could suddenly hear the half finished scream too. His next scream was his first breath, and he was fully pink and well toned, and covered in sticky vernix.

The cord had pulled tight around his neck, and I was very glad when I saw it that we hadn't messed around taking pictures of the unburst sac. The cord was only long enough to bring him to my lap. It was too short to slip over his head, so I just unwound him like a spool.

I wasn't sure what to do next. He didn't seem that interested in nursing. I felt worried that allowing him to nurse would contract my uterus in a way that might disconnect the second twin's placenta. We sat peacefully for about twenty minutes until I felt annoyed by the sensation of his cord between my legs. I took that to mean it was time to cut it.

Normally, I would deliver the placenta before separating it from the baby, but there was so little slack, he would be in the way of the second delivery.

After about an hour, he started to root on me but that seemed to stimulate labor to resume. I wrapped him up and handed him off, and stood to deliver the second twin. My contractions were quick, short, and gentle, and a very small amount of blood started to dribble from me. My husband was videoing this time! I reached inside hoping to feel a head, and instead felt a collection of bony things. I hoped they were arms, but I eventually unhooked and pulled one down and out, and it was a foot.

I allowed myself one full second to completely panic in my head, and then forced that part of me to go silent. The heard inner instruction that he would stop at his head, and that it would be okay and to keep forcing myself not to panic. I knew that you weren't supposed to touch a breech delivery, but my hands did not allow that to happen; I pulled out the other foot, took hold of his ankles, and gently started to draw him out. There was more blood streaked on his body the farther out he came, and I had a sense that my shrinking uterus was starting to pinch off the placentas.

One he was out to the waist, I just started supporting his weight with my hands, and one last contraction pushed out his chest and arms. As was stated, he stopped at his head, and when I tried to push there was no force in my baggy deflated stomach. I had more inner instruction screaming NOT to push, not to move, to relax completely, and that if I didn't I was risking causing nerve damage.

In the next moment, I heard my husband's name in my head, and just as I was about to ask for help, he tossed his phone aside and jumped up to help. He worked his hand inside me over the baby's face, so he could push his fingers out to make a little air passage to his nose and mouth. I was not aware that this was his plan, and it took all my attention to keep myself in a state of relaxation and suppress the panic.

Once the air passage was secure, he waited for a contraction to expel the baby's head as my uterus shrank back down and I regained stomach muscles. Then I had a flashback to a video of a breech delivery I'd seen on YouTube, where the midwife tilted the baby downward to face back down the birth canal. That unhooked the baby's chin and rolled out the back of it's head, so it could be pushed out easily.

I told my husband to do so, and as he did, his fingers followed the baby's face back up my birth canal. He said he felt a rush of fluid and blood over his fingers, and he said to me 'it's okay, I have his face, he has air," When he said that, I immediately realized we were at the finish line. I gave a tiny push, and the baby flew out into my husband's arms.

He handed the baby right back to me and grabbed the phone again to resume video. Right as the camera focused on the baby, he spat out the mouthful of blood and fluid that had rushed down over his face. He was also bright pink and breathing steadily, though his muscle tone was relaxed, much like my singleton was at her birth. He cried a little after we sat down, and I wrapped him up too.

My second twin, due to the crammed space in my uterus, has a mild condition called torticollis - a bent neck. The ligaments on his right side have taken months to stretch out and straighten, and he's still not quite there yet. Perhaps if I'd been over-anxious about getting his head out it would have injured his neck, which was straightening for the first time in his life.

The placentas were delivered together about forty minutes later, along with some considerably sized blood clots. They were joined together by the second twin's empty sac, but they were not touching and appeared whole and complete. I felt a little weak probably mostly from the blood loss, but otherwise fantastic. These were the first full, complete breaths I'd taken in months, and I finally felt like I could eat. We did it! 38 weeks and 3 days, each boy weighed five pounds and a few ounces, and both were in perfect condition on arrival.

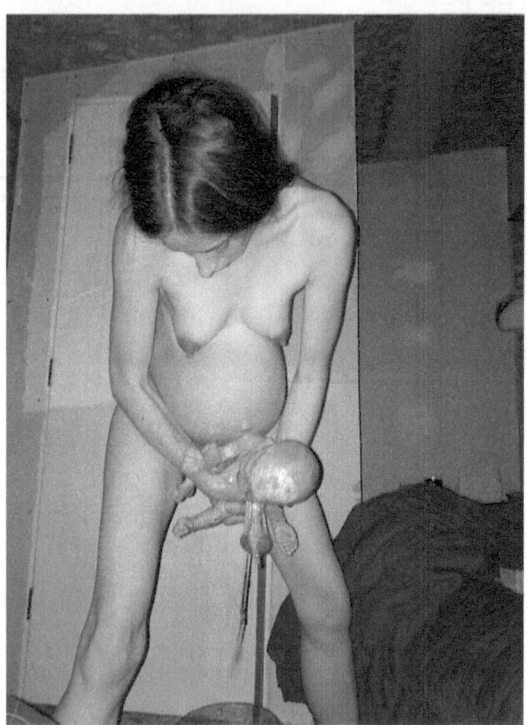

Twin A, born head first

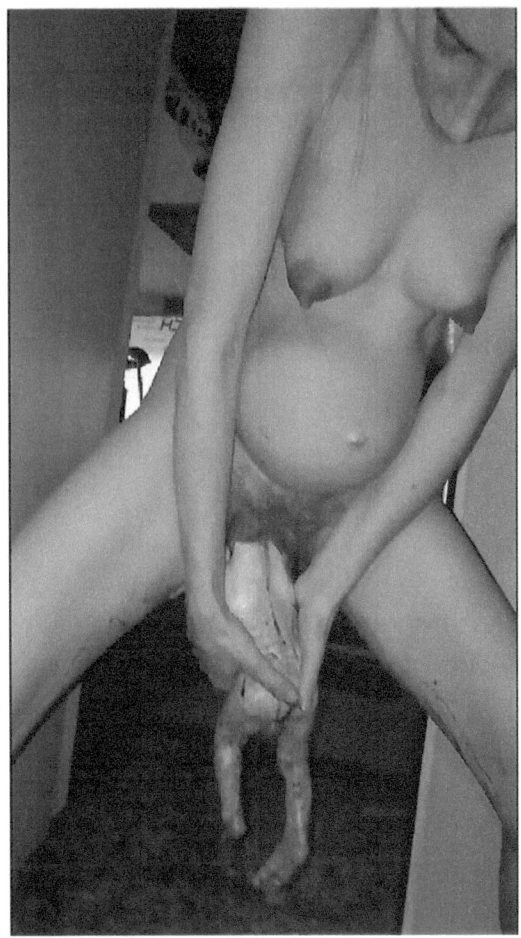

Twin B, born breech

Freebirth Miscarriage and Stillbirth

THERE ARE MANY OUTCOMES to birth. We all hope for a living, perfect baby. Sometimes, babies are born sleeping. Heavenly Grace shares her story of her son, born sleeping at about 11 weeks gestation. She chose to freebirth him. Here's their story. Pictures follow and may be difficult to view for some individuals.

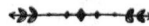

The Birth of Arrow
Submitted by Heavenly Grace

ON FEBRUARY 26TH, I went in to receive proof of pregnancy, since I had been UP (unassisted pregnancy). Besides one independent ultrasound at 9 weeks, the OB decided to do a scan. I should have been just over 13 weeks but baby Arrow was measuring 11 weeks with no heartbeat. My husband was in the car with our girls, so I left in a hurry without discussing my "options."

We already knew we wanted to free birth Arrow so we went home to wait. By March 18th I decided we needed to look into cytotec so that we could still try for a freebirth before any OB declared us "too much of a liability" to prescribe it.

On March 19th, at 5 p.m., I took my first two pills orally and contractions started pretty fast but stayed steady with no bleeding or discharge by 8 p.m. So, I took the next two pills and within minutes the surges were much stronger and consistently 5 minutes apart.

Our bereavement Doula arrived just after 9 p.m. and kept me company chatting in between contractions while my husband snoozed on the couch. Poor guy drove me 5 hours round trip to get the cytotec that day.

By 11 p.m. I had to stop talking/listening completely during a contraction and close my eyes and breathe and remind myself to relax every muscle. Around 11:30 p.m., our Doula got a call that her daughter was rushed to the ER, so she had to leave.

When she left we moved to the bedroom and I felt most comfortable standing and walking, and during each contraction I would squat next to the bed and hang off the edge of the mattress and shove my face into the bed while my husband gently rubbed my arms and upper back.

I believe that's when transition really hit because I texted a sister in Christ and told her I couldn't think through contractions anymore and asked her to pray for me.

Right at midnight I felt a huge contraction, squatted down, and when I stood after the contraction felt a GIANT gush of fluids that filled my super pad front to back instantly.

I panicked for a second thinking, "Was that blood?!" I moved to the bathroom and my husband stayed in the room as he doesn't do well with blood. I pulled my sweats down and immediately could see there was hardly any blood on the pad, and there was my sweet baby, Arrow, laying on my pad.

I instantly picked him up and laid him on a chux pad and my first thought/action was to move his little leg and check his gender. I cried, "I have a son!"

I had heard during loss baby is usually born in their sac this early so that's what I was expecting, but instead he was born in a gush of waters like so many full term freebirths I've read about.

After I had checked him out, I felt another contraction hit and knew the placenta was trying to deliver. I expected it to be small and easy. I started the tub, took the rest of my clothes off, and got in. I opened that bathroom door and asked my husband what time I ran to the bathroom, and he said, "Twelve, why?" And I said, "Because I delivered our baby and wanted to know what time Arrow was born."

He immediately ran to the door and asked me if I was okay and I said, "Yes, but I need to deliver the placenta. I'll be okay." But then another contraction hit and it was so much stronger than any I had during the night previously. I hit my knees and ended up squatting in the water, I reached down and could feel a bit of the placenta right there.

Another contraction hit and I yelled, "Jesus help me!" I could feel FER (fetal ejection reflex) working its magic with every contraction, so I breathed and relaxed to let my body do its work.

At this point my husband came in, despite the tub full of blood, and I immediately unplugged the tub so he could refill it. As it was filling back up another contraction hit, and I felt the urge to push with FER and the placenta delivered into my hand. It was so much bigger than I expected. I put it on the chux pad next to arrow and took a deep breath. I did it. I really did it. I brought my baby earth side all by myself. And my next thought was, I CAN do this full term next time.

After I cleaned up, I started inspecting the placenta to make sure there were no obvious missing pieces. The mother side was out, so I flipped it to the baby side, and there was Arrow's cord insertion, and my feeling about twins was suddenly and unexpectedly confirmed. There was a perfect 5 week gestation sac attached right next to the cord insertion. There was a tiny dot inside that was confirmed to be a 5 week embryo. We named Arrow's twin Cedar. I was honestly so scared to give birth to my sleeping baby, but it was such a healing and empowering experience. I'm so thankful we got to freebirth the twins.

Unfortunately, my Doula was going to take labor photos, and since she had to leave, I don't have any. But I took lots of pictures of Arrow and some of the placenta and Cedar as well.

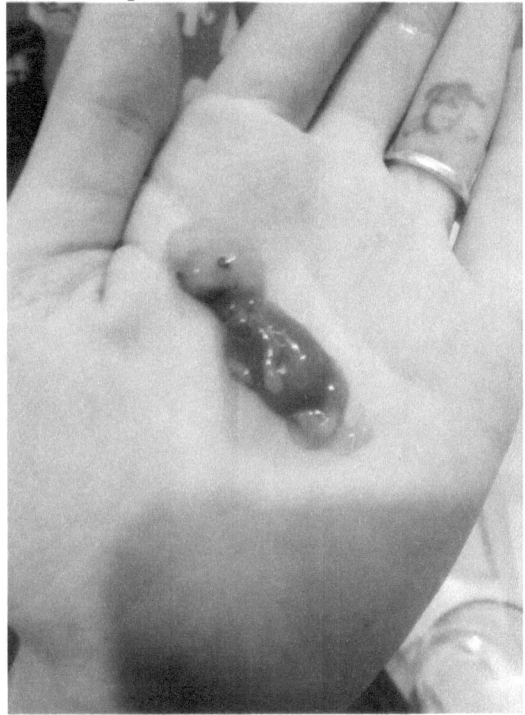

Arrow, in Heavenly's palm

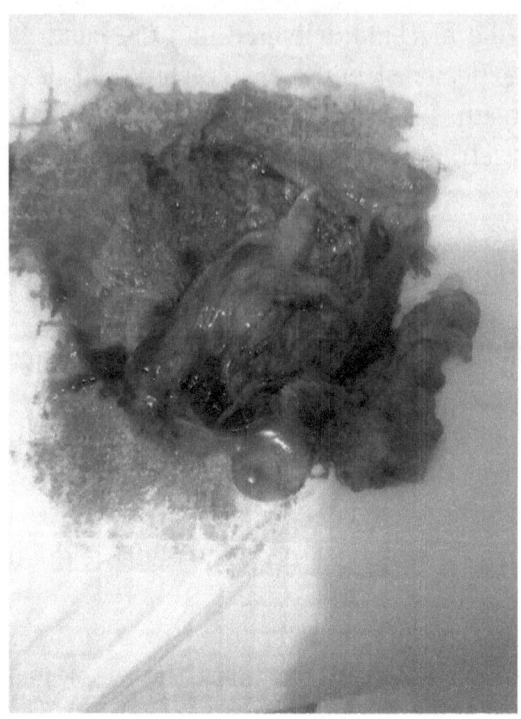

The placenta; the tiny, clear sac at the bottom is where Cedar, Arrow's twin, gestated.

Freebirth Transfer to Assistance

SOMETIMES A PLANNED FREEBIRTH includes a call to a midwife, a phoned ambulance, a change in birth location, and medical personnel at a birth. These stories are crucial to understand as one journeys to freebirth. Read without judgement, open your mind and heart, and examine the feelings that come up for you. There is a time and a place to intuitively seek further care. I hope that these stories will aid you in making the decisions you make as you embark on a journey towards birthing free.

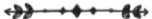

A Post-Birth Hospital Transfer

Submitted by Laura

BELGIUM

I started having mild contractions in the afternoon, but didn't know yet I was in labor. I was at exactly 39 weeks gestation, and I had been having Braxton hicks contractions since week 30. It felt just the same but slightly painful, just like a period pain. I ignored it and kept on tidying the house. We had planned to spend the night in my mom's, and when I realised I might be in labor I thought about seeking advice on an online Freebirth group to know whether to cancel our plans or not. Well, I didn't ask, and I decided to trust my body instead. This was my first baby so I probably still had quite a while to go before the birth.

My partner had to get hemp from the shop, so we decided to go to my mom's after he got back. Although I hadn't been timing the contractions, I couldn't deny that they were getting stronger and closer, and I wasn't sure anymore about going to my mom's for the night. When my partner was back, I told him I'd actually rather stay here and asked him to make dinner.

When dinner was ready, I had to breathe through each contraction. I stopped eating halfway through and started to walk about. When my partner realized I was in labor, he left again to go to the nightshop (as soon as it opened, so it was 9 p.m.) to register the new SIM card to be able to phone an ambulance in case we would need emergency help, and he left me alone with the cats.

By the time he was back, I already had my bloody show and was vocalising through the contractions, so we decided it was time for him to set up the birth pool. I went in for a shower because I got sick all over myself. I believe this is where my water broke.

Then, what messed up everything: my dad arrived, and as soon as I was out of the shower, he was phoning an ambulance. A few minutes later, two firefighters were here. I was then laboring in the pool. I suddenly thought I wouldn't make it, and that I would need an epidural, and I kind of felt relieved my dad phoned the ambulance.

A few contractions later, a wonderful baby boy was born.

Right after the birth, the firefighters wanted to clamp the cord, thinking baby would die if they didn't. I really had to insist for them to wait until it stopped pulsing, and they pulled out the placenta right away after that (they were even about to call the police to have a witness in case one of us died. They really didn't have a clue).

Then, a bunch of doctors arrived, and I unfortunately made the mistake to let them convince me to transfer to hospital, which I very much regret. They gave my son the vitamin k shot and eye drops without telling me (I found out 4 days later), and wouldn't give our placenta back, which I had asked for.

I didn't have an unhindered birth as would have liked, but I am glad at least that my baby came earth-side before any doctors came.

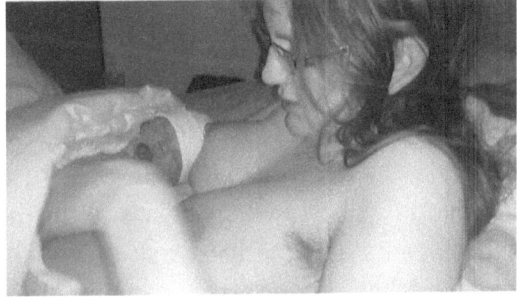

Intuitive Transfer from Freebirth with Twins
Submitted by Natalie Holden

AUSTRALIA

Birth, as anything in life, is unpredictable and full of surprises. It tests your limits, challenges your perceptions, and if you let it, changes you in ways you could never have imagined. I have been changed in ways that I can see in the mirror, but the more profound change is not so directly visible.

After having two unmedicated hospital births that were great but left me wanting (one induction, one breech which I fought for tooth and nail), and an incredible powerful freebirth, of course I was going to freebirth the twins I knew were growing in my womb long before I had physical evidence. Seeing two wriggling babies on that grainy black and white ultrasound screen at 12 weeks was not at all surprising to me. It was a big relief though to learn that they were dichorionic diamniotic (di-di, where each twin has their own amniotic sac and placenta and the least risk of complication), as in the weeks prior I had had a few worries about mono mono twins changing all the plans I had for my pregnancy and birth.

At first I did explore other options for the sake of my husband. Was there an independent midwife whom we could hire? No, not within a 3 hours drive. Could I return to hospital, a stronger and more confident woman than the last time I gave birth in hospital, and fight for a low intervention birth? I knew I was capable of fighting, but I didn't want to have to go through my pregnancy and labor prepared to battle at every turn. And if I did beat the odds of the 80% cesarean rate for twins at my local hospital, the most positive hospital birth falls far short of the way birth was designed to be. So no, freebirth was the only option.

Later in my pregnancy I did compromise with my parents in agreeing to birth at their home in town rather than our place in the country. If they felt more comfortable with me being half an hour closer to the hospital in an emergency I felt that they would be believable to support me without fear. My parents' home was still a place where I felt comfortable and at ease, and as a bonus I would be able to pre-set up a birth cave in their spare room, something I would not have had the luxury of doing in my own home.

My pregnancy progressed uneventfully and without medical care until 32 weeks when I chose to make contact with the local maternity clinic to request an ultrasound to ensure the placentas would not be a hindrance. I told them I did not need anything else from them, and thankfully was never contacted for further appointments.

My babies were healthy and my belly grew and grew and grew as the weeks passed. I had felt since the beginning of my pregnancy that I would give birth between 38 and 39 weeks. My feeling had been spot on with my first two girls, but my son surprised me over a week earlier than I expected. Even so, I got sucked into the "twins come early" mentality so prevalent in our society.

When I reached 34 weeks, the gestation I felt comfortable freebirthing from, I breathed a sigh of relief and assembled my birth kit in my van so I would have everything I would need should I labor so quickly I wouldn't be able to get to my parents house.

When I reached 36 weeks the "I can't believe you're still pregnant" comments increased exponentially. For the first time in pregnancy I felt so over it. I didn't want to rush them but I hoped they would be ready soon. I was so uncomfortable and chasing after my toddler was practically impossible.

At 37 weeks prodromal labor started. Every evening contractions would start up that made me wonder if I would have to head to town that night. Almost every day I was going to my parents house and hoping for some sign that labor would be soon and I wouldn't have to drive home.

From 38 weeks I was certain labor would be happening that week. Once or twice the prodromal labor contractions were strong enough that I actually texted my photographer to be ready for a call. But I never did have to make that call.

The Sunday I was 39 weeks I couldn't face the thought of going to Church and facing the awful litany of "why aren't those babies here yet?" So I didn't.

I did, however, go to church on my due date. Not many have the opportunity to say they are due with twins *today* and the ability to make such a claim amused me enough to want to tell people Besides, I was going to be pregnant forever so there was no point in being a hermit.

After church I went for a beach walk with my dad, his dog, and my three children. A steep set of stairs down and back up after a 2km walk on the beach surely was going to put me into labor. I was done. My belly could not possibly grow any more.

I was going to stay at my parents house until the babies were born. Retreat into my cave, all decorated with affirmations, Bible verses, and pictures I had colored, and not come out until my babies were born.

I was so looking forward to this birth. Not only to meet these beings growing within my womb. Not only to experience that thrilling oxytocin surge. Not only to breathe and roll over and walk without pain again. There was definitely a part of me excitedly looking forward to having an epic, powerful birth to share. I joked that my births kept "one-upping" each other. From unmedicated induction to hands off vaginal breech, to a fast freebirth to a twin freebirth, any future births surely would almost be a let down.

The evening of my due date my husband was going to go back home to our farm but before he left I insisted on a quickie in the hopes the prostaglandins might kick things off. He left and I went to have a bath, envisioning myself having my babies right there in their lovely deep bathtub.

I began to feel surges. Unlike the prodromal contractions I had been experiencing for weeks these were popper surges that gripped my belly tighter tighter tighter and only released when I felt like I couldn't take it anymore. I counted for a while 6-8 minutes apart and lasting 70 seconds.

The intensity had quite a ways to go still I knew, but I also knew that once my surges reach the intensity that I know to be active labor I don't have long to go. So when do I call my husband back? He's only just gotten home. I'll give it a little while.

I put on my satin robe, turned on my fairy lights and Spotify playlist and started rocking on my birthing ball. Melting into the surges and relaxing myself into labor land with my breath. I didn't quite get there. I alerted my photographer that I would be calling her likely some time in the night and called my husband to come back. I resumed laboring in the peaceful stillness of the night, butterflies of anticipation fluttering in my tummy.

When my husband arrived I asked him to massage my lower back as I was experiencing a fair amount of back labor by then. I could tell it was still the early stages of labor so we decided to go watch TV in the back bedroom for a bit. I was able to lean over the birth ball while watching TV and my husband kept massaging my back. If I couldn't focus on the TV any more then we would have felt like active labor was super close, called the photographer and returned to my birth cave.

It was nearly 2 a.m. when I sent my husband to bed; it was looking like this labor was going to take a while, and I was going to need him to be well rested. After a while I decided I should try to sleep too. I hoped to be able to get an hour or two of rest and wake up in active labor, hopefully while it was still dark.

Sunlight flooded the bedroom when I woke up at 7 a.m. the next morning, super discouraged to have slept through. I got back on my ball, bouncing and rocking and hoping to bring the surges back. And they did, but weakly and far apart.

We agreed that hubby should go to work in the meantime. My parents fortunately had some time off and we're able to watch the kids all day while I tried to bring the surges back stronger. Something must be off with baby As position. This was very unlike my usual labor pattern, and with the back labor I had been experiencing I decided to spend the day working on getting the babies into more optimal positioning.

I went curb-walking around my parents neighborhood, lots of lunges, rocking on the birth ball. I looked up the Miles Circuit and did a couple rounds of that. When my husband got home from work I had him do some Rebozo sifting with my ring sling. It was exhausting and my labor pattern through all this was sporadic. I could go a couple of hours without a single surge, and then a couple hours where they were 10-20 minutes apart. But despite all my efforts, the length of time between surges was only increasing.

I was so discouraged when I went to bed that night. I nearly sent my husband to the store to get some castor oil. We talked and prayed together, and decided that if labor still wasn't progressing overnight in the morning I would have my dad drive me to the hospital for an NST and to find out what position the babies were in. I knew that was what was holding labor off and felt that if I knew exactly what positioning twin A was in I would be be able to encourage baby into a better spot.

Morning came without a single surge, much to my dismay, so after my husband left for work my dad drove me down to the hospital where I steeled myself for the battle I knew was coming.

The midwife I saw was really lovely and supportive, asking consent for everything, including asking if the doctor could come in and examine me and do a bedside ultrasound as she was not at all sure what positions my babies were in from palpating. She reminded me that the doctor was likely going to make recommendations that I would not agree with, but that they were only recommendations.

Doctor G came in with the portable ultrasound machine, the same young female registrar who I had seen 8 weeks prior. Even with ultrasound she was having a really hard time to figure out where they were lying and asked for permission to do a vaginal exam. I was 4 cm dilated and she could feel a spine. That was most unexpected. I was prepared for one or both of the babies to be breech, but a transverse (or more specifically a sacral oblique) presenting baby had never even entered my thoughts.

I know babies can move all throughout pregnancy and even labor, but full term twins with the second twin down so low on top of the first? It seemed impossible that either would be able to move out of the way enough for a vaginal birth to be possible.

The suggestion of course was for an immediate cesarean. I knew that was not necessary. My babies and I were healthy and strong.

There was no emergency. There were still things I could try to help get the babies moving. I called my husband so he could help me be strong and calm me down, because even though I knew what I needed to do the doctor's words, though spoken compassionately, shook me to my core.

When he came we went for a walk down the corridor and I broke down sobbing in his arms. Once I had calmed down and cleared my mind we returned to the birthing unit to let them know we were declining the cesarean and would be going home. We left without signing the AMA form, and with a promise that I would be in touch the following morning, or if anything changed in the meantime.

I called the only Webster certified chiropractor in out region but the earliest she could see me was two days later, on the Thursday. I made the appointment anyway. She would be successful, she had to be.

Before returning to work my husband took me back to my parents house and did another rebozo session, this time inverted and sifting my bottom instead of sifting my belly on hands and knees. I could feel twin two move farther away from twin 1, hopefully giving enough room for twin 1 to be able to move as well.

That afternoon Doctor G phoned and asked if I would go have a better ultrasound so we could have a clearer picture of the placental health. I knew she was looking for a reason to convince me there was an emergency, but I agreed anyway, hoping to see evidence that the Rebozo and breech tilts and inversions I had been doing were already making a difference.

Within a couple of hours I was at the ultrasound, and twin A had indeed moved - but not for the better. Instead of being sacral oblique with feet up at the face my baby was now fully transverse with a leg bent backwards, toes pointing out my cervix. Still, there was hope that this meant they could get themselves situated more ideally.

Later that afternoon, Doctor G called to discuss the ultrasound and I could not stop rolling my eyes at the predictability of every tactic she used to try to convince me that my placenta (singular) was failing, my babies were showing growth restriction measuring at 3% when they had been at 25% at 33 weeks. I told her that I understood her concerns, but I did not feel similarly and I was still going to keep trying to get them to move and wait for labor.

While I was still hopeful that the babies would move I did begin to prepare myself for the possibility of having a cesarean. I sought out positive cesarean stories, particularly where they weren't wanted, and listened to a few on the birth hour podcast that I found particularly beneficial. I phoned my sister and asked her to share her cesarean birth stories with me.

The hospital phoned a few times on the Wednesday morning. I ignored the first few phone calls, wanting to ignore everything going on and connect with the babies and encourage them to turn. But they were persistent in trying to get a hold of me so I eventually answered, declined to go in for a cesarean and articulately explained my reasons for doing so when asked.

I told her I was not satisfied that that was sufficient evidence that they were not thriving, stating the unreliability of growth estimates, especially as they had been done on different machines by different techs, and the earlier measurements were hastily done as the sonographer knew I wanted to keep the ultrasound exposure below 5 minutes.

Doctor G agreed that ultrasounds are notoriously inaccurate at estimating size at term, but stated that it's the only measure they have for determining health. I said that wasn't a strong enough indication that babies weren't healthy, and I trusted my intuition better than technology. Though I did agree to go in for a NST that evening when my husband got off work.

I spent the rest of the afternoon doing more inversions and breech tilts, and basically hung out in frog position for the day, praying for babies to turn and intermittently crying.

I met my husband at his work at 4:30, we quickly did another Rebozo and made our way to hospital.

We ended up being there for a frustrating 4 hours because they kept being unsure they were picking up both babies separately and spent ages with the ultrasound trying to make sure they were getting two different heartbeats as they kept measuring so closely in sync. While I kept implying that I had enough and wanted to leave, I never said the actual words, "I'm done and am going to leave now," until nearly 9, which I should have done after the first pointless hour.

My kids were asleep when we got there at 9, only the second time ever in their lives I wasn't there to put them to bed, and the first time they didn't even get to say goodnight on the phone.

We had a bite to eat and my husband went to bed. I had a good cry and spent more time in serious prayer. Not just that the babies would turn but that I would have peace about it if they didn't.

As soon as I went to bed around 11 p.m. I had a strong surge. And then another. I got up and labored quietly alone for a little while, wondering how long I should labor to give them the most chance of turning before going in. But since only a couple hours before baby A had been footling transverse, I hadn't yet had any chiro, and hadn't felt any shifting movements in the meantime, I had this sense of peace flood over me that this was it. The babies had chosen their birthday, but also a mode of birth that I had not expected. And while I was afraid of the actual surgery itself I had no doubts that it was what my babies needed.

I woke my husband and my dad was still up and went and woke my mom. With a sense of complete calmness I went about packing a suitcase - totally haphazard. I didn't have much at my parents house in the first place that would have been good to take to hospital. I did have a wave of sadness when I went to grab baby clothes from the basket and realised I didn't have anything with me that didn't say "born at home." I told mom she would need to go shopping for a couple of outfits before coming to see us in the morning.

The four of us prayed together, I kissed my sleeping children, and I phoned the hospital to let them know we were coming in and off we went.

Halfway there I realized I had forgotten to insert sterile gauze in my vagina for microbial seeding before we left the house. So I did it in the hospital parking lot.

We called to let them know we were there, as a midwife has to come down the front door after hours. Meanwhile I was still having powerful surges maybe every 3 minutes that were taking focused breathing. I was meditating on my affirmations during them "I am strong and unafraid,""God is my refuge and strength," "God has not given us a spirit of fear, but of power and of love and of a sound mind," were some of the main ones that came to my mind. But most of my affirmations I had hung up in theology where I intended to birth I found were easily transferable to preparing me for the cesarean. Even "the only way out is through."

I was hooked up to the CTG upon arrival, and they needed to do an internal exam so DH removed the gauze and put it in a ziploc. I had been 4 cm at the two previous checks, and was now 7 cm at 12:30 a.m., an hour and a half after my first contraction.

I was gowned and stockinged up and given the pre-op meds while waiting in triage for the surgical team to arrive, and then wheeled in the bed down the hospital to theatre. My husband was with me up until the point that i went into theatre so he was there when I met Patrick the anesthetist and my nurse Tracy. The anesthetist was asking me a bunch of questions while I was contracting, which I answered by shaking my head yes or no. Then we had to say goodbye while DH went to get gowned up and I went into theatre.

Getting the spinal wasn't as bad as I thought, and I immediately started going numb and had to have help laying down. The anesthetist used an ice cube to confirm that I had no feeling below my breasts, and once the drape was up and I was shaved they brought my husband in.

I had previously discussed with the Doctor (Doctor L the registrar was the one we had seen earlier that evening, and the Doctor who did the surgery) that we wanted delayed cord clamping and the babies would be laid between my legs for a couple minutes before being taken to the warmers, and then brought to me for skin to skin within a few minutes. But it suddenly occurred to me that I had never asked to keep the placentas, which I said to my husband. The Doctor overheard and said that would be no problem.

My husband joked in the theatre that with my varied birth history we are trying for "the complete set", and a waterbirth VBAC next time will finish it off. Everyone laughed, I think probably rather surprised to hear us joking about the next birth while I was being cut open.

Then I could feel painless tugging, and a sudden weightless feeling and I knew the babies were out. My husband said our son has a brother but he hadn't seen the other baby, and when we asked they told us she was a girl. I could see her from the warmer she was taken to, but his warmer was out of sight behind the drape. She was huge and healthy and everyone was exclaiming over how big they both were.

My son was brought to me for skin to skin right there while they sewed me up, and I said he was so tiny. I was sure he was my smallest baby. From across the room my daughter just seemed so much bigger. She had had meconium in her waters so they wanted to observe her on the warmer for a few extra minutes. And then I began to have a reaction to the anesthetic. I felt light headed and began dry retching. Patrick recovered my blood pressure quickly, but I still felt kind of yuck and out of it for a while so my memory is kind of hazy afterwards. But I remember Patrick and hubby walking to recovery beside me and we were there for about an hour.

I got skin to skin with my daughter, and apparently tandem breastfed but have no memory of that (but I have a photo). I remember that I kept drifting in and out of sleep. I so badly had wanted to be fully present to be able to take in and remember every small detail of the birth, but hadn't considered the effect the drugs would have.

When I could start wiggling my toes and moving one of my legs Patrick bid is farewell and we were wheeled to the maternity ward.

Babies were born at 1:31 a.m. (same time) both weighing 7.5 lbs (same weight within 5 grams). We got to my room around 3:30 and there was a spare bed for DH to sleep on, and we both crashed hard til 7.

The babies were with us the whole time.

I stayed four days in hospital and my kids, who had no preparation for me having a hospital stay did absolutely amazing with the transition. I was especially amazed at how well my 2.5 year old adapted. My mom brought the kids in to visit twice a day and we face timed before bed each night.

It was far from the birth I was expecting, and I do have some sadness about what I missed out on, but it was still a positive experience that has left me feeling powerful and amazing. And I know it's because I retained my autonomy and was treated with respect throughout every decision making process. Something that I so dearly wish every woman could say bout her birth. Birth is unpredictable, messy, raw, and takes us to places we never thought we would have to go, but we all deserve to feel powerful and amazing no matter how we give birth.

I may have been cut open, but I still birthed intuitively and autonomously and advocated for my babies as best I could with the knowledge I had at the time, and that's something to be proud of.

More Freebirth Stories

"I'm very drawn to stories about ordinary women who do extraordinary things."
–*Rachel Weisz*

Ezra's Freebirth
Submitted by Laura Christensen

THIS PREGNANCY WAS SUCH a beautiful and spiritual journey. It was especially important to me because this birth had been planned in my heart for almost two years. The experience my first born and I encountered at a hospital was both traumatizing and robbing of what I envisioned birth to be. I made a promise to myself that day that I wouldn't let that happen again.

When I got pregnant (with my second), I started diving into stories and advice from other women: how their labors went, variations of what it looked like, how they felt, influences of who was present, if and why they transferred, etc. Initially I thought, "Oh, of course I want a midwife, just in case." But I challenged myself further: what was that "just-in-case" if I wasn't in a hospital?

It surprised me when I learned what the routine procedures were of a midwife and legally what they could and couldn't do, also having the power to transfer women against their will, which is one scenario I came across frequently. They are bound, just as doctors are.

I began feeling uncomfortable at the thought. I knew I had to protect myself in my vulnerable state of labor, being not physically able to tell anyone no when they offer advice or demand action.

The number one thing that other free birthers told me was always the same though, "Listen to your instincts. They will tell you what to do."

It all started on the afternoon of Tuesday, August 6th. That's when the contractions began. The *REAL* contractions. They were every

10-20 minutes, and it felt much better to lean over something and relax while they happened. Wednesday I had the "bloody show", which was exciting considering I thought this "early labor" was going to last a week long. Thursday, August 8th, I had a doctor's appointment for a "non-stress test" since my baby boy was measuring small, just as my first born was. Because of this, the doctor had given me the "pep talk" once again on how I should just be induced, to forcefully bring my baby into this world because if he can get fatter faster out here, why keep him inside?

In my heart the whole time I knew he was perfect. I knew drugs were not the answer and not the way to birth my son. My instincts and God were telling me he was fine. I declined his offer, again, and asked him to sweep my membranes instead (separating my bag of waters from my cervix), in hopes that it would really kick me into gear. I started contracting immediately afterwards. OB also said I was 3cm and my bag of waters was bulging outside of my squishy cervix. He gave me his cell number and said to call him when we got to the hospital, I said "okay" and left.

We got home by 3:00 p.m. The contractions were about 4-5 minutes apart and were strong. At 5:30 p.m. they were about 2-4 minutes apart so as I sat on the living room floor leaning on my yoga ball I was trying to eat food and chug a green smoothie. I asked Preston, my husband, to fill the bathtub for me. He was watching football and was getting pretty anxious that this could be it. My sister called me, and I didn't want to answer since I couldn't talk during rushes. She then immediately called my husband, who also didn't answer. Then we both got missed calls from my mom. Shoot, they knew what was going on. I was trying not to let their anxious energy get to me and stay focused. I did not want ANYONE knowing I was in labor. My state of mind was beginning to alter at this point, and I was focusing more intently on myself. Surrendering to my body, repeating my favorite birth affirmations.

When I finally got in the bath it was about 6 p.m. It felt amazing. I was getting a little anxious thinking "this could be it, my baby could be born tonight!" so the bath really helped. I had my computer playing this one birthing affirmation video which was my calmer-downer-get-in-the-zone video pretty much throughout my entire labor. I prayed a lot too. The water definitely slowed contractions, that or it dulled the intensity of them.

I was really tired for some reason and kept falling asleep as I was leaning over the edge of the tub. Eventually, I got out. It was 8:00 p.m., and I felt so much better. I felt "prepared" for labor, physically, mentally and spiritually. My water hadn't broken yet so I decided to check my cervix and see how dilated I was. It felt like 4 or 5 cm, although I didn't want to be too intrusive since putting anything inside during labor increases risk for infection. I used two of my urine analysis strips to make sure I wasn't positive for protein, and I used the stethoscope to listen to Ezra's heartbeat. It was 130, which was 10 bpm higher than it normally was. Contractions were about 7/8 minutes apart or so at this point and I thought, "Crap, I shouldn't have been in that bath for so long."

I was starving so I got dressed and went downstairs. Husband was hanging out with our daughter and said he made dinner if I wanted some. I tried to eat some chili but ended up just having a few bites and a huge glass of chocolate milk. I couldn't help but think, "This is probably going to come right back up very soon."

The kitchen was a mess so I decided to do the dishes. By the time I was done it was around 9:30 p.m. It was now clean and peaceful and dark outside. I was so glad I made it to dark because birthing at night is what I've envisioned my whole pregnancy. I had my vanilla candles lit. I walking around the dining room in the darkness and leaning over the counter during rushes rocking my hips. What I thought was really neat was that my hips/pelvis sort of crunched when I rocked back and forth, I'm assuming it was my pelvis being open and relaxed, ready for baby to pass through. Our bodies are so amazing!

Anyway, nothing was more helpful than walking and/or standing. I'd have Preston come over during a couple rushes and squeeze my hips together, which moved several inches! Again, so fascinating! But it felt like relief. I thought how thankful I was that I was at home, because in a hospital there's no way I would be able to relax like this. By 11:00 p.m. I was super exhausted and just wanted to sleep but kept thinking "No, I'll just wait it out. He's gotta be here soon!" Preston was trying to put Jade to bed cause she was being a little rebel, and I was sitting on my yoga ball in our bedroom hanging onto the side of my dresser. Rocking back and forth and groaning/moaning during rushes.

Once Jade was down I asked him to go get me food cause I was starved again. I figured I wasn't in transition yet, so I'd quit stalling and get some energy in me! He came back with a cut up orange and mango and ice water. I was eating between contractions then stopped to hang back onto the furniture during. At this point I thought they were 5 minutes apart again, and thought, "WHEN will this pick up and I'll know I'm closer to having this baby?!" I tried checking my cervix again and was thoroughly disappointed when I thought it felt the same as it did hours earlier. Preston was tired so he fell asleep on our bed.

I decided I'd try to sleep too at this point since I had no idea when Ezra would be born. I sat on the bed with three pillows on my lap so I could just lean over and rest my head. It kind of worked but then I'd wake up to a seriously intense rush and since I was sitting still, it SUCKED. I decided I should just get back in the bathtub. By this time it was about 1:00 a.m., and I was thinking, "Am I really doing this right now?! I am crazy." I had my phone and called Preston to try to wake him up to come in the bathroom with me and tell me I could do this but he didn't wake. After maybe an hour I got out and wanted to try sleeping again. It worked for another 15 minutes maybe then awoke to a deadly contraction. I checked his heartbeat with my stethoscope, which was still 130 bpm, then got back on the yoga ball.

At this point I was definitely in a different state. I was repeatedly acknowledging my body's work. That I wouldn't get in the way of it and that the intensity I was feeling was just a sensation. It really helped. After awhile I was trying to get Preston to wake up because I needed him and his support. After a few yells and kicks he woke. He was hugging me as I was rocking on the ball and it helped a thousand times. It's amazing how much comfort and love affect everything. I was groaning pretty loudly at this point and knew it wouldn't be long until he came out. I started shaking and going from hot to cold, kept telling Preston to take my sweater off, and put it back on, to open a window, and then to shut it.

I remembered this feeling of shakiness and knew I had made it to transition! I told Preston to run and get me a bowl cause I'd be puking up everything in my stomach soon. He did. I puked; only three times though. I kept saying, "There's soo much pressure," and Preston said I should get off the ball because I was, and I quote, "blocking the hole" for the baby. (Ha ha).

It was probably 2 or 3 contractions after that that all of a sudden my water broke, popped actually. I immediately stood up, and the fluid poured out of me as I dove for the floor, on the shower curtain and puppy pads we had laid out. HE WAS COMING. I was kneeling with my face buried in our bed (our bed is on the floor) groaning "EZZRAAAAA!" so low and so loud I thought every neighbor was going to hear me and be worried. Contractions switched up at this point and became short and close. It felt like they were 15 seconds of my body pushing him down, then 1 minute of peace, then repeat. I remember thinking, "Thank the Lord I'm not anywhere else!" My body was doing this, ON ITS OWN. It felt so powerful! I was just there along for the ride, and it was such an incredible feeling. One that will you will only ever know once you experience it. With each contraction, I was getting more and more excited and each time it felt like "this would be it" But it wasn't.

I noticed I was sweating profusely and thought that was really neat, just because my body was working so hard to get him out, and yet I wasn't forcing myself to do any of it.

The last two contractions (out of maybe 15 total since my water broke) I finally reached down in hopes of feeling his head, and it was there about to come out, then went backwards again. I knew that's how it worked, like two steps forward, one step back, but I felt he was ready, so I actually "pushed." His head came out! After 13 hours of labor.

Preston said, "His head's out, and his little hand!" (Nuchal hand) He told me to push again. I waited for another contraction, and once it happened I pushed a little bit. "His shoulder is out!" he said. (THAT was a crazy feeling) I breathed a little then pushed more, and the rest of his body came out, which finally felt like relief.

Time had stopped at this point. I was instantly hit with euphoria. I DID IT. I birthed my baby. I reached down and snatched him straight from his hands...I was squatting now, resting my butt on my heels and tried to put him on my chest, he wouldn't reach. He wasn't floppy at all, but he was coughing out fluid and sounded raspy. I felt for his neck to see if the cord was there (because it was dark in our room). It was. I tried hooking it with my finger but it was super tight and wrapped twice, so I laid him down on the amniotic fluid covered floor (next time I will have towels down on top of the puppy pads because there was A LOT of fluid) and unrolled him like a little potato, then scooped him back up.

In these moments I'm not sure if it was all instinctual or my memory suddenly renewed, but every piece of information I studied, what to do about the cord, what to do first, second, and third if they aren't breathing...All of it became SO clear in my mind, like I was opening up this giant beautiful book of feminine wisdom. I put his chest on my hand and tilted him down to drain the fluid from his lungs, then once he sounded better I cradled him in my arms, he was SO tiny.

I sucked on his nose to get any remaining fluid out, but it was clear. He opened his eyes and looked up at me. He had no vernix or blood on him, just perfect pink, warm, wet skin. I was rubbing his back and telling him how much I loved him and how glad I was that he was here. Preston grabbed blankets and towels to cover us up. I looked up at Preston and said, "He's soo small. You should call the paramedics."

He said, "Why? Is he okay?" and I said "Yes he's fine but he's like 5 lbs!" So he did. I'm not really sure why I had them come, honestly. If I waited I would've changed my mind, but he was so small it shocked me. I spent the whole pregnancy praying for an 8 lb baby and when my little nugget arrived it shocked me. They arrived after 10 minutes or so.

They were nice and respectable. The woman firefighter told me, "Wow, you're so brave!" They basically just listened to his heart rate, looked him over, said he looked great, small but great. They had the sterile utensils to do the cord, and since it was white and limp already, I cut it and they clamped it for me.

They had me say, "I decline to transfer," to some woman on the phone who sounded snotty, but fortunately that was the only negativity I encountered. They wished us well and left after about 20 minutes. He was indeed tiny, but perfect. Perfect in every way.

Once they left I gave baby Ezra to Dad, after he had laid down sheets trailing to the bathroom for me (so much blood!) so I could go jump in the shower to clean off, go to the bathroom and try to deliver the placenta. I got in the shower after failed attempts on the toilet and squatted. Finally, I could go pee! The placenta followed and came out. It was small, like Jade's had been. I forgot to get a metal bowl beforehand though so I just set it on a towel on the ground. Then I climbed into bed and Dad gave me back baby, and we snuggled. Then we called our families to tell them the good news. After that we slept a good six hours, woke around 9 a.m., and I had my husband make me a huge breakfast. It was beautiful and perfect in every way.

The Tale of Thea Evelyn
Submitted by Laura Christensen

SMALL BACKSTORY:

Since Ezra (my second child) was young I had this feeling/vision that we would eventually have another baby someday, and she'd be a girl. I also always had my heart set on Luna. Some days I'd sit and cry wondering when it would be the right time to have this little girl join our family. Thinking it well could be another 10 years away or I was just daydreaming so hard and that there never would be another little girl.

After a year of baby talk with hubby, I surrendered. "Yes." The time could be now. I could envision another baby. She was conceived the next cycle. The whole pregnancy felt like I was living a dream I was so unsure of it, even pushing it away thinking it was just fantasy. I doubted myself. Was I disconnected? Why wasn't I having these strong intuitive feelings? It was different. But when we found out she in fact was a girl, it all felt right. Why would it be anyone else? It was her.

Saturday (Estimated Due Date, March 31):

It was a full blue moon, and after filling Easter eggs with my hubby and debriefing him on labor stuff (for the first time this pregnancy), we went to bed. He fell asleep, and I snuck outside to stand under the full moon. It was cool and windy with a clear sky. I smiled as I watched my wind chime sing me a song. It was something I had wanted to buy to put outside my window for when baby was born. Something I just *needed*. I talked to my baby, telling her I was ready when she was, but that she could take another week or two if she needed. I was in NO rush. I reaffirmed that she would be born when she was ready and it would all be beautiful and perfect. Singing praises to my God for this miraculous healthy being that had blossomed in my womb.

Monday, April 2nd (40w + 2 days): I startled awake to my waters releasing at 3 a.m. It was flowing fast and paired with some strong contractions. "I knew it!" I told myself. The night before I was so busy and had this constant nagging feeling of "GO LAY DOWN, GO REST," but it was Easter so the day was full of family events and I ignored it.

I got up to go the bathroom and ahh…that sweet, distinct smell. I grabbed towels to lay down on the bed, a red one between my legs. I remembered Maryn Green saying you can see the specs of vernix in fluid. I looked and I could see. My body felt full of excitement and anxiousness. Oh my gosh I am so close to her, but yet still felt a world away. I tried sleeping until around 10 a.m. but had butterflies hardcore. Waking to maybe every other contraction, and eating occasionally then going back to sleep. I finally decided to face reality and time contractions around noon. 4 minutes apart! There went my denial. After that I had a super big contraction that released a TON of fluid. Need to drink more water, I thought. I swear I must've released a gallon or two by now. I spent the next couple hours in the shower, eating or just hanging out.

I felt emotional, I wanted to feel and cry and I couldn't really. It was very odd. It was Monday afternoon, sunny (I preferred night time). I was, in a way, trying to avoid labor until nightfall. My husband stayed home from work and my kids stayed home from school. I remember thinking I'd really like some coffee and a target trip right now, but I'm not risking either of those. 4 p.m.

I texted my bestie to say come over after work. I decided I wanted her there for loving support for myself and for my husband and kids as well. She arrived around 5:30 p.m., and at that point I was in the bath. I loved having her there with me because she kept me calm. We chatted and I ate like four chicken thighs while in the tub. I felt kinda like I was toggling between places. She grounded me mentally, and she was also drawing me from a place I could've easily floated away to. After the tub she watched the kids so me and hubby could get some intimate time. I had never craved or felt so dependent on him in my entire life. It surprised me because my last labor I wanted to be completely alone. But this time, he was my comfort.

The night went on. Dinner, hung out outside. Basically, mentally, I was stalling labor. I was trying to just float by and avoid anything crazy. Like how some women just hang out and oops, here comes baby! The kids were loud and distracting. It was daylight. I still felt funny. Silently waiting for the peace of the night. Finally around 8 p.m. the kids were put to bed, the sun was going down, and I thought, "Okay, now it's go time." I made a green smoothie and had a contractions that brought me to my knees in the kitchen. Bath time again. I started feeling nauseous and shaky and knew transition was near.

11 p.m.

Got out of the tub and made my way to my bedroom. Transition had been going on for at least an hour at this point, and it was real. I felt like an animal as I needed to prepare my spot to birth. I had this corner in my bedroom all decorated with Christmas lights and birth affirmations, towels stacked high and everything ready to go. During my pregnancy I had thought, "This will probably be my birth space." It felt warm and glowy and cozy.

I thought how freaking epic it is laying out my supplies for the second time in my life. Unsealing the packaging for my herbal tinctures. All the towels, the scissors, the bowl. I layed out the shower curtain on our floor and felt it slip around. "No way." I tossed it aside and tried a small area rug (to save the carpet) with towels over it. "No." This wasn't working. This wouldn't be my spot. I had my husband there now, and I started getting really vocal. Leaning on and hugging him, trying to get relief from the exhaustion.

My legs were burning from fatigue like I had been running a marathon. The yoga ball, the bed, on all fours. I was hot and cold, shaky, and throwing up at this point. Baby girl was ferociously punching me with her fists, and for at least a good hour straight she did this. I remember thinking, "Poor babe she's probably fighting to get in a better position." (She came out facing my thigh, by the way.)

I was hungry and sent hubs to go get me fruit. What seemed like 27 hours later he came back with this beautifully decorated plate of cantaloupe and bananas. I think my exact words were "Where the f*** did you go?!" because it felt like he had been gone for eternity. I ate some fruit but immediately threw it up.

At some point I was alone in my room again, and I knew I needed a nap. The nausea slowed, I knew laying down that I might wake to a contraction that would rock me, but I NEEDED that nap. I layed on my side, closing my legs and feeling like I'd just shut some medieval gate (not kidding) *boom* and slept. I don't know if it was one minute or five or ten, but I got it. I woke up as my husband walked in the room again and I suddenly felt her move down. I shot up and immediately started roaring/moaning.

"The floor," I tried to say but couldn't really talk. I needed to be grounded. This was it. Wow! Birth is so powerful. I asked for help waddling to the toilet because I NEEDED to poop. Got to the toilet. But quickly realized I didn't need to poop poop, I needed to poop a baby. I started basically yelling at this point during waves. She was moving down, and I could feel her. Literally, the most insane feeling ever. I reached in to hopefully feel her head, and it was quite a ways up. Shoot. I thought to myself. This is why I decided not to do checks this time.

I dove for the floor since my husband was worried about her falling in the toilet. I somehow managed to move in front of the shower so that he could be behind me to catch baby. I was sort of on all fours but squatting. I grunted and yelled as my body pushed her down. Between contractions, I was able to rest and breathe, getting a break from the intense feeling of a baby in my vagina.

The pushing, though. It was different this time. I had my best friend in front of me. I was holding onto her with my husband telling me baby was "right there." With each contraction now I felt myself stretch, then she'd retract as it ended. "THEA!" I yelled out her name. Again and again and again. "Come on baby girl, come to me Thea!" I needed her. This unknown child was now suddenly missed and longed for. It was maybe three or four more contractions and by the last one I roared harder than I ever have and POP. Out came her head. Relief!

Hubby said, "c'mon mama bear, push!" I waited, I breathed. "Push!" He said again. "Shush!" I said in my head but physically could not speak. Finally, another contraction, so with it I grunted and pushed/my body pushed, and there went the shoulders. My husband grabbed her as her body emerged. She let out one loud cry. I turned over and he quickly handed her to me.

"You did it mama bear!" He said. I wanted to cry, but I couldn't. I was too high. Too relieved, too happy. Sitting there hugging my baby. I could hear some mucus so I sucked her nose and mouth with mine and spit it out on the floor. She had dark hair!

I sat there hugging her thinking, "Oh my gosh I did it." The hardest thing I've ever done to date. I could not even describe the relief. I was just so happy. So at peace. I got up and walked to our bed. We sat there staring at her, smitten over all her little features. Jade snuck in and I welcomed her over to meet her baby sister. She was so in love. (Later she told me she heard me pushing Thea out, and then she heard "a little cry." Then she waited some more to come in the room. Her level of consideration brought me to tears.) I was on Cloud Nine.

After 20 minutes or so I felt the placenta was ready to be born, and I couldn't stop moaning through the contractions. I tied her cord and cut it, she actually cried, and that threw me, like what in the flying hell? I handed baby to dad while I got in the warm shower to birth it into a metal bowl. I was so cold, but the shower helped warm me back up. I squatted, peed, and birthed the placenta. Now I was ready to cozy up in bed with my baby and enjoy this pure form of ecstasy. I laid her on my belly and laid back. She did the breast crawl and showed her efforts for trying to latch on right away. I helped her, and she nursed for over an hour! We later woke up Ezra to show him his baby sister. We couldn't contain the excitement. We laid there for hours before I could actually sleep. High as a kite with my new beautiful baby now on my belly. My hubby got me Gatorade and food, and I laid there feeling completely happy and in love.

This is birth.

Total labor time (from waters breaking) was 21 hours, and she was my biggest baby yet. 6 lbs, 13 oz. 19" long and a 14.25" head!

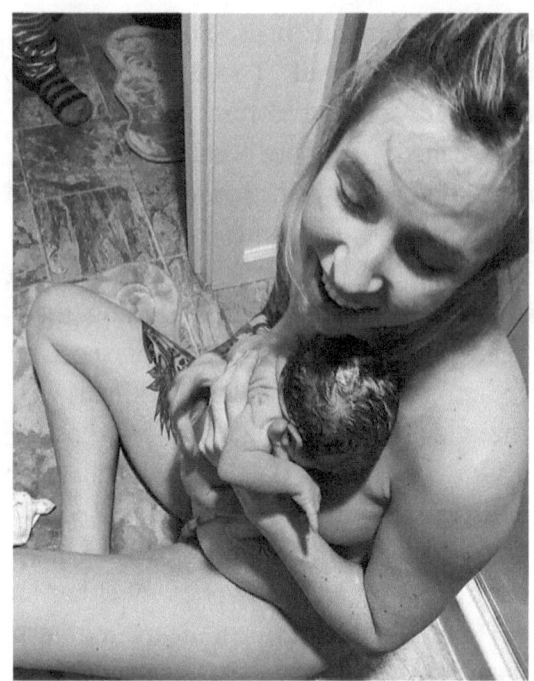

Birth Like Breath
Submitted by Anonymous

ONE OF MANY IMPORTANT steps to having a joy-fueled life is to release all unnecessary fears. As a woman, fear of birth paralyzed me in my ability to enjoy making love with my husband. I was always afraid of getting pregnant, not enjoying my pregnancies, and having to "risk my life" to birth the baby. There was a lot of fear there.

I knew that was not true in the deepest parts of me, but the fear programmed into me needed proof of what my heart was telling me. So, I went on a search for women birthing alone in civilization due to their dissatisfaction of assisted births with a midwife or doctor at home or in the hospital. At this point, I'd already had five home births with a midwife, and they were not what I had hoped.

I was petrified of birth after five home births…Even more than before, and at no fault of the midwives. They did everything they were taught and forced to do, mostly because their licenses depended on it. They were obligated to interfere with birth way too much, which caused problems. Instead of tuning into their intuition, they were tuned into fear of the worst and if anything went wrong they would blame the birth itself, just like doctors do. In my further research, I discovered that wild people of the earth who give birth without interference have experiences that are as smooth as taking breath, and yet our systems and advanced ways in medicine are supposed to make "civilized" childbirth so much better…Right!?

If that is true, why is it we are suffering so greatly in this process? The only reason we think modern medicinal practice is best, is due to deep programming about the way we are to perceive the birthing process, while being encouraged to repress our sexuality and accept a life where being unloved, unprotected, and nutritionally deficit has become the norm.

Birth is as easy as breath; that's how creation designed it. Well-meaning people have been interfering with nature's perfection as the world around us fills our heads with so many un-truths and taboos. I've known for some time in the deepest parts of me that they were wrong. I went through a lot before I was brave enough to challenge common perspective and the current standard practices involved in the birthing process. Thanks to my mentor Laura Shanley, I finally did it!

I challenged my fear, and I conquered it. I did it despite being told I was too old, had birthed too many babies, that I was "high risk," by well-intentioned but completely disconnected people (doctors whose views and training were deeply rooted in fear about birth.) I was having serious dis-ease within me. My life needed a major change so I could heal. I was told by the doctors that I was wrong in my thinking about childbirth and healing, but I knew better and refused to buy into their stories. Later I was able to prove them wrong, of course. I was healthy, my heart was just broken. I needed to change my mind about how I was seeing things in my life and remove a few major toxic unwanted things, and that's what I did.

I had two unassisted births despite everything they told me. It seemed like everyone around me was doing their best to scare me, but deep down I knew they were all wrong. I also knew they wouldn't listen to me as they truly felt the information they were offering was in my best interest. But no one knows our bodies better than we do, so I graciously listened to their advice, ignored them, and did what I knew to be best anyway.

I came to understand the reason why my previous births had been such nightmares. One was that I had invited people into my sacred birthing space who carried deep fear-filled energy about birth. And, to add insult to injury, I was paying many of them to be there. I too was in doubt and in fear back then, and I let all their BS influence me for way too long.

Here is the story of my recent birth. After this experience, I would never ever do it any other way again. It was my best of seven births, and I did it alone. It's like they say: if you want something done right, do it yourself.

The wild birth of my sweet son Willow Love was just him and me in my bathroom, lit only by my Himalayan salt lamp.

I was very anxious to have this baby! My brain was on strike and my pelvic bones had been killing me for months, to the point where I refused to move unless absolutely necessary. I was really scared and concerned the pain would prevent me from having an efficient labor, so I decided that the most important thing I could do during my labor was to constantly remind myself that if I was in pain, I needed to go through it, and the more I allowed the pain to be without resistance, the quicker the baby would come out. So my first priority was refusing to hold that baby back, no matter how much pain I would be in.

Secondly, I had to relinquish the concern about the baby coming out breech. I was a breech butt-first baby but have not had a breech, and at the last ultrasound this baby was sitting, so naturally, I was anxious. Instead of feeding into this, I worked hard through any fears imposed on me from others about breech and decided that if that was the way the baby was coming, I was ready to have that experience as well.

My due date was September 4th, and I went into labor on September 1st, a little early as I had hoped. My daughter calculated it for the 1st so Willow came to us on his due date or perhaps a little early. Either way, I was happy it was happening!

I had gone to bed late, around 12:30 a.m., and after resting for a few hours woke to period like cramps, which was kind of alarming considering out of 7 births I'd only had this experience with my first UC attempt where I labored for 72 hours! Not an experience I want to ever have again!

I wasn't sure what was going on but the cramps kept coming, and I finally decided I should get up and see if this was really happening now. I went to my pink bathroom where I had all my birth supplies and where I would birth and labor. I sat on the toilet to pee and see if there was any mucous coming out, as this is always my sign of labor, but there was nothing. The cramps kept coming and strong. I couldn't do anything but breath through them.

I decided to go ahead and set up the camera and supplies just in case. The contractions I had were really uncomfortable on the lower half of my uterus, so I got some oil and began deeply rubbing it into the muscle, which did give me some relief. I also decided to get in the tub as I waited to see if the cramps would subside or if this was the real deal.

In the tub things kept coming on strong! I was conflicted for a bit at first because every contraction felt pushy, but I kept hearing other people in my head saying you don't want to push until you're fully dilated, blah blah blah!

I listened to these imposed thoughts filling my head for a short period of time and then suddenly remembered that those rules don't apply to me! My perspective was not those of any of those people, not my family, my friends, or any doctor. According to my rules, I was to listen to my body and it's cues only and forget the rest.

Simple, with every contraction I would push to the level that my body was asking without being over strenuous.

After a while in the tub I needed more ice water, so I got out, dried myself off, got dressed and went out in hopes to not wake anyone. Having had several strong contractions I brought a chux pad to contract on in case my water broke or mucus came out. At this point still no mucus plug, so I was very confused, but the rushes were so overwhelming I forgot to be concerned about whatever I was concerned about. This was a great thing. It's never helpful in life, especially during birth, for us to go into that energy space of worry. I got my ice water, came back and labored some more in the bathroom. It was super intense! It seemed like all the things I was doing before had stopped helping, so I decided to go get the wine to see if that would help.

While in the kitchen I could not find the wine opener! It was only lit by my salt lamp, so I could not see very well, and all of the sudden I noticed a wiggling sensation on my feet. I turned on the light to see a bunch of little weevils on the ground! OMG! What!? I'm in serious freaking labor! Hahaha! Really? I had just detail-cleaned this kitchen four days before (they came from the glass recycling that's supposed to be clean, but one of the babies had put food in there).

I knew I could not clean them or leave them either. So, who's the best person to wake up to help me that won't kill my groove? I settled on my 9-year-old daughter, Trinity. She's very calm, sweet and soft. I quietly woke her and she cleaned up the mess, made me juice and had the wisdom to decide on her own she'd better leave me alone because she could see I was working hard! She brought my juice and said, "I better go back to bed now." Of course, she went in the room, woke up my 12 and my 6-year-old, where they eagerly waited to hear the baby's cry.

While Trinity cleaned up the bugs, by some miracle I found my pocket knife that had a cork opener. I opened the wine while having a bunch of super intense rushes! Hahaha! I poured a bunch and went back to the bathroom. I downed as much as I could. I was sure I would puke, but I didn't. I had more and more intense rushes, so I drank the rest! The more I drank I would relax for a second, but that would bring it on stronger. A good thing.

I now needed more ice water. Why didn't I have Trinity get me more? Oh well! Off I went to get more when I saw my husband awake in his room, so asked him to get it for me. I went back in the bathroom and things were coming on super strong now, and finally mucous plug! Exhilarating joy came over me. Then my water broke, hahaha! Now I knew it was happening and close.

My husband came in to give me the ice water, and I grabbed it. I did not want him near me. All I could do was push him out and close the door. In that moment I was having strong rushes one after the other. I was in the middle of a strong rush, and that's all I could do. Several more contractions and I felt up and could feel a hard head. Baby had turned a few days before, which I suspected because pelvic pain was less on the right side where he had been sitting for months and was now even across my pelvis, and the hard ball by my ribs was gone, too.

A few more intense contractions then one huge, long, super vocal rush where I was in a leaning back squat hanging off sink position and baby's whole head and body came spinning out of me in a single giant push! I had not intended for that to happen! Hahaha! It was out of my hands. Nature and creation knew what was best and took over. He was out! I did not expect that.

Baby was crying and pink and wiggling. I wanted to lean forward to pick him up, but I could not move! My vagina was throbbing like crazy on fire! I was very vocal about it.

My husband could tell I was close when I kicked him out of the bathroom and stayed outside the door. When he heard the baby's cry and me being pretty vocal about my vagina throbbing, he came in and I asked him to wrap the baby in a towel and go get me an ice pack to help my vagina chill out. He came in and gave me frozen raspberries. I asked him to pick up and hold the baby because I could not. The ice helped a bit but not enough. I could still not sit back. What I really needed and wanted was my herbal ice pack. Thank you, Jesus, I had made those! I sent him for that, grabbed the baby, and while I waited I began feeling the cord. I could feel it pulsating! I've never felt that before. My husband returned with the herb ice pack and that did the trick quick! Thank God! Instant relief! Herbs are amazing! Thank you herbs and free nature given medicine.

I was now finally able to sit and hold my baby. At that moment, I felt so happy, excited and in love with this baby! (Something I was sad to not have felt with my first unassisted birth. I was TOTALLY numb! I realize now it was because of the horrendously heart-breaking relationship I had with my husband and family.) Now I was getting all the lovely rush of emotions that they say you get in birth.

I knew that to get the placenta out I needed to engage my muscles by myself. I leaned forward and stood up on my own. I immediately felt the placenta flop down to my pelvic floor from the top of the uterus where it was all pregnancy. A very cool feeling that I'd also never felt before! I grabbed the placenta bowel, stood over it, pulled gently on the cord (okay to do because I knew it was no longer attached at all), and eased it out. Ahhh, that felt so much better! It was all flattened out from so much baby in there! There was much more blood then with my first UC but nothing serious, I felt great. I think I was a little drunk from the wine, hahaha!

The blood was grossing out my husband. He's a wimp about body fluids; I'm like whatever! I ignored it and asked him to clean it up. I had the tub still filled, so I decided to get in to clean my self and baby up a bit. I had the baby in my arms still attached to the placenta, and trying to hold both was too hard. I no longer felt any pulsating (in the cord), so I tied it off and cut the cord, leaving a long part still on baby. I stayed in the tub for a bit, washed off, etc. and then I got really hungry.

All three of us went to the kitchen. I decided I would rather make my own food and have my husband hold the baby. Butter bread with organic Raisin Bran cereal with raw milk. I told H to get baby dressed while I ate, thinking the kids would wake up when he went in my room to get a diaper, but nope, they were pretend sleeping! Little sillies.

I decided to go to sleep in my husband's room to not wake the kids so I could get some rest (not knowing the kids were awake and eagerly waiting this whole time).

Baby and I laid there and breast fed on one side for 20 minutes. That's all baby wanted, all he wanted to do was sleep! Birth was so peaceful for him he did not realize he was born. He slept through the whole labor and the whole next day! I realized later that he thought he was still in me being fed by the placenta. Haha! Little silly!

While I rested in the room, my husband was finishing the clean up, including the placenta. I asked him to put it in a glass dish with lid and freeze it. I suddenly heard a loud noise and knew he had dropped it! He was covered in my blood! Hahaha! Really funny! Paybacksies for him acting like a psycho the week before! Luckily, all that was lost was some blood, so I'd prepare and consume it later.

After a while the kids could wait no longer and came out, We cut the rest of the cord with the kids and made a heart out of the extra cord. All the mucus plug that had not come out in labor was all stuck on the top of baby's head!

Of course none of us could sleep. I was so pumped I texted everyone in the family and Facebook announced, too! I felt so good my sister and mom came over and brought us food. Yum!

I realized later that I felt so good in part because baby would not eat and just wanted to sleep, so I was not having any after birth pains. As soon as the evening hit, baby realized he was starved, not being auto-fed by the placenta. I nursed him all night and the next day. I was so delirious the next day from no sleep, but still soooo pumped! I was just rambling incoherently at that point.

Willow's cord fell off at 4 days old, and he was 5 days old when I wrote this. He was born around 9 lbs+ on September 1st at 3:25 a.m. It was a 2.5 hr labor start to finish and all caught on video.

Funniest part of my birth was my 17 year old son had friends sleeping over that heard the whole thing! Hahahaha! They came up in the morning to find me with a baby, filled with joy, acting as though nothing had happened because nothing out of the ordinary had happened. Birth is as natural as breath, just like the wild hunter gatherers of the earth show us.

Eleven Pounds and Freebirthing
Submitted by Anonymous

YACURUNA STORM CAHUAYA ANDERSEN
December 13, 2017

After weeks of prodromal labor and being seven days past due, I gave up all hope that it would ever happen. I caved a bit and went to get evening primrose oil four days before his birth. I was breaking apart 4 capsules and putting them up near my cervix, figuring it can't hurt to help things soften up down there. I'm not sure if it even does or did anything but I'm a doer, and it helped my brain chill out a bit. On day three a creamy, white, good-sized glob of boogery stuff came out, but nothing else happened. I was so sad! Then again, the day after that, more globby white stuff with minimal cramping came, but when I got in the tub the cramping stopped. I woke up the next day still pregnant!

At this point I was really annoyed! I was almost a week past my due date and baby was more than well done! I just could not believe it anymore. I also did an unassisted pregnancy. I'm not at all an amature, this is my 8th pregnancy and my 4th unassisted pregnancy, 3rd and a half unassisted birth. I know how to do pregnancy and birth. I was 100% certain on my due date, having on-point periods and keeping track of my periods very closely, I knew when my last one was. I knew the exact day I conceived. I was way past due! I did not care about all that 'there is no exact due date' stuff anymore; I was miserable! Having been in prodromal labor for at least a month before this was killing me! I'm a single mom taking care of 5 other kids, running a business at the same time, though thankfully my business is from home. I worked really hard through pregnancy to build it up, and I had established it well enough by then that I could mostly chill out and roll with this. But I still had a lot on my plate with taking my kids to school and back, to their dad's and back, dealing with their behavioral issues, groceries, homemade meals, cleaning, renters behavioral issues, etc. I was barely making it. In addition being 41 yrs old, couldn't this baby just be born early?

That day I had mild contractions on and off. I was determined that night had to be the night. My daughter said, "Wouldn't it be funny if you woke up pregnant?" NO! NO it would not! I jokingly disowned her as a daughter in that moment. I went to bed, boys asleep all around me, my daughter and her friend asleep just outside my door in case I went into labor. We share the large living room area turned into our room so I can rent out our rooms, it's my way of keeping my kids safe and with me.

At 2:45 a.m. I started contractions. I laid and observed for about 15 minutes to make sure they were legit this time and they were very strong and consistent. At last! It was time to go to the bathroom and check for any signs of mucous bloody show, etc. Sure enough, there was bloody show mucus! As I was wiping, my water exploded right into the toilet! WOW! I was shocked! I have never started labor that way! My water would always break when it was push time with all the others. OMG! This is go time! How fast was this moving!? I was so excited! Leaking amniotic fluid with a towel between my legs, I snuck back to my nest to birth the baby. At last!

Back in my nest, I pulled out the doggy bed where I planned to birth my baby. It was already lined with chux pads where I stood to labor, breathing through every contraction and setting up things I might need in between, but not much time was available in between! Things were super intense from the start. I got out my massage vibrator thing which I used to massage the sore areas when I'd contract in front of my belly, my sides and my butt. The best idea ever! It felt so good! Where was this at all my other births? I was so tired, I just wanted to sleep. After all that waiting it was finally happening, and all I could do was wish it would hurry, or stop so I could sleep.

Not too long into it Leonidas (5) woke up and he was so excited that it was happening! He was talking to me, telling me to "Push, Mommy!" etc., then my other two boys Willow (3) and Mason (6) woke up as I was getting more and more vocal. Really loud! I couldn't help it. It was sooooo intense! The other two joined in on the coaching, haha! Commenting "Eww," on every drop of stuff that came out of me. "Eww, mom is pooping, Eww mucous, Eww blood." etc.

It was all on chux pads, and I would remove layers as I'd soil them. They would all tell me to push, and it was not push time, haha! About 40 minutes into it I tried to call baby's daddy a few times in Peru, he did not answer. I tried, but it was too hard to keep calling, so I decided I'd record it for him instead.

I kept laboring with the boys. They were so excited, talking to me and to each other! I did not want them waking anyone up, so between contractions I'd tell them, "shhhh," the best I could, and that's about all I could get out until another one would come, literally back to back! I started to feel freezing. It's a thing that can happen when one is in transition, so I asked Leonidas to put my socks on, I literally could not do it. He struggled and struggled but it was too hard for him. I had one sock on only halfway, and I could do nothing about it! Hahahaha! I could barely catch a breath in between contractions. When I tried to laugh a hard contraction would come. I was laughing on the inside! I'd heard my son Bobo (9, that's his nickname) wake, and he was in his bed playing on his phone at that point.

I called him over to please help me put my socks on, so he reluctantly did. My sweetest child. By the way, in our house birth is treated like breath. It's a normal, 'life is happening' thing here, and all my kids have been around birth and birthing. We bathe together, etc. To them it's all normal, "Oh, mom's giving birth again, okay, whatever."

I got my robe on and kept laboring. I felt up my vagina with my finger and I could feel my baby's head right there, about an inch inside! He was so close! I was freezing and contraction pain was brutal. It was taking an enormous amount of force to get this "little" one out. All of the sudden I heard my renters dog making noise.

"Crap! He's going to wake her up!" Of all the people, I did not want her to wake up, so of course she did. A concern I had was them noticing I was in labor and calling the ambulance due to their ignorance, fear, etc. about birth, but as hard as I tried to get a place to rent to birth away from home, I could not get one. The funds were just not available.

So there I was, laboring with five unpredictable renters in my house. I guess everything happens for a reason, whatever that reason was I'm not sure yet. I heard her get up, my mother also woke up, the girls were up, everyone was now up because I was so darn loud! When my mother peeked in to see how I was doing, I told her, "I'm fine, but will you please take the boys?" They were so cute and I hated to kick them out, but they were very distracting and hard in that intensity of labor. I also sent my daughter Trinity and son Bobo to call in my renter. She said if I needed any help to call her, and since she was up, I did.

I was in so much discomfort, I just needed a little bit of relief. I asked her if she had some greens, but she did not. (A very helpful thing in my other solo births.) Since she was already in my room and offered to help me, I asked her if she could massage my upper butt with my magic wand massager. I don't think that's what she had in mind when offering to help me, but it's what I needed. Haha! This woman has totally medical, fear-based beliefs about birth and everything, so it was just too funny! It felt sooo nice! But I was so freezing my teeth were chattering, and I was shaking so badly I could not get a grip on it. I asked her if she would fill the tub for me with hot water, so she did. I just wanted to put my feet in to warm up. I walked past the kids and friend to get into the bathroom, and I closed the door behind me. When my feet touched the water it was so nice! I just got completely in the water. Ahhh, sweet relief! Instantly, the freezing went away and the pain was totally gone!

I had a few moments break when my baby's head starts pummeling out of me! I reach down and holy shhhhh! Oh my God! He's HUGE! He's going to tear me to shreds! I hesitate. I stop pushing, which stopped his movement out and with that the contraction completely halted! I can't! I CAN'T! I have no other choice! There's only one way out! Regardless if he tears me to total shreds, I have to get him out and I have to get him out that way. That's the only way out!

Right away the next contraction came, I control-pushed and screamed as his emergence to outer earth ripped me apart to the fullest I could be! I used my hands to help wrap my vagina away from his emerging head! I was left quite wide open, beaten, bruised and battered but not torn to shreds. If I tore, I don't know. It felt like at least some good skid marks, like a rug burn down there. I did not look. I used my ointment and frozen herb pads. It took a bit to heal and pooping was not a fun party. I had to hold my bits together down there when I pooped with hemorrhoid and it was frightening. But, after some time my lady bits healed up back to perfect! I sell the ointment I used to heal my lady bits in my shop right on this web page in the Healing shop if you're interested.

I'm in the water with his head out of me, totally under the water, an unplanned water birth. I'm waiting for the next contraction to get the rest of him out when my renter comes back in the bathroom! I forgot to lock the bathroom door! What is she doing in here? She brought towels. Now she's freaking out about his head being out under water and is telling me what to do like in the movies. She tells me quick put your feet up here and pppuuussshhhh. Hahaha.

So now I have to be a teacher with a baby's head between my legs! I said, "No, I'm not putting my legs up there, and I'm not pushing, no I'm not doing any of that. The baby is fine, just relax, I have to wait for the next contraction."

It's so interesting how a grown woman who has birthed I think 6 babies herself does not have the slightest clue about how to really give birth. That's what happens when you're not allowed to really birth your own baby. Not her fault.

A few moments later came the next contraction and all 17.5 inches of his HUGE shoulders came out! One shoulder at a time, then the rest of the giant baby came sliding out and he was out! Sweet relief! I let her grab him from between my legs and hand him to me.

He was floppy and not responding, and it was a bit hard for me to want to focus after all I'd been through with life stuff beyond what I've put in this story, pregnancy and now super intense birth of a HUGE baby! He is limp, I'm exhausted, my renter in there freaking out now that he's limp and not immediately breathing. No relaxing for me, now I have to calm and teach her more about how he's totally fine, sometimes it takes a few minutes for them to react, breathe, etc. blah blah blah. He is and will be fine, please go away and shut up, you have no clue what you're talking about, this is not a movie! (I did not say that I just thought it.) Haha!

Of course, I was NOT thrilled that he was not breathing right away, but it was what it was, freaking out was not going to help, keeping calm and doing what I needed to do calmly was, and I was rubbing him on his back with him on my chest.

I felt and the cord was still pumping blood and oxygen to him very strong. My renter was still freaking out that he was floppy. I reassured her more that he was fine, that the cord was feeding him oxygen. With that I knew he was 100% fine. It took a few minutes, but he started reacting and pinking up a little bit at a time. It took him a total of 3 minutes to start to breathe, calculated from the recording. Again, I did not worry at all to give him mouth breaths because his cord was still pumping very strong, I knew he was getting all the same life giving oxygen he was getting for the past nine months through his pulsing cord. He was a HUGE 11+lbs, and he just got pushed through a very tiny hole. I'm 5'1" and my down there parts can't even handle a large penis, so….

I understood he was in a little shock for a moment after all that, and at the nine minute point he started to cry, cord still pulsating. The water was so so nice we just chilled there for a while. It was so comical because the water was also red from the normal amount of blood that comes out at birth, and my renter seeing me sitting there perfectly content, "Nope, we are not moving. We are chilling here in our blood bath for a while," was hilarious! She was left traumatized, I'm sure of it. But I did not care. I was cozy and comfortable, it was so warm, and my baby was out and breathing and doing great! I was in bliss. The kids came in to see their baby brother and were grossed out about the red blood in the water. I told them it was just red color bath colors, a thing we regularly use, so they would relax about it. They did not believe me.

After a while I decided I wanted to get the placenta out. I was getting strong afterbirth contractions, and I was sooo uncomfortable.

I got up in a squat to see if it would just come out in the tub, but nothing. I could feel that the placenta was up at the top where it had been. I decided to go to my bed to see if I could massage it a bit and dislodge it. Getting out of the tub while holding a huge baby was a bit painful, so being that my renter was there I asked her to lend me a hand to get out now. She'd already seen all my naked lady bits. It was so annoying she was there, but it was also helpful. (She ended up getting paid for the help she gave with a month and a half of free rent.)

When I got to the bedroom, I felt to see if the cord was still pulsing in hopes it was not so I could cut it. I wanted to be free of baby to work on the placenta if I could. It was giving me so much pain with more huge contractions. I really wanted it out and to know I was done done! Luckily, it had stopped pulsing, so I let my renter who followed me into the room cut the cord.

She was so excited about having seen his birth, having "caught" him, "delivered" him as she tells it. A wee bit of an exaggeration, but for sure having been there for the whole thing. I was so happy to have him out I let her have the honors. It was really cute and cool to see her joy in what she was doing, and for sure a super cool thing to be a part of. She took the baby to show him off to his brothers, sister, and friend. The cord was so long it reached all the way to my feet! I got on the bed to massage the spot where my placenta was and immediately I felt it was gone from that spot. I stood up and felt up there, and I could feel it right at the vagina entrance. Success! I could get it out now!

Knowing it was totally detached from the uterus, I pulled gently on the cord and pushed with a very painful contraction and torn up hurting vagina, and a giant placenta came out with sweet relief! Almost the same size as a small baby! It was born into the dog bed, the place I had planned on birthing Yacu. At least I got to use it, and boy did I, I labored there as well! I got my frozen herb pad in place inside my depends diaper (way better than pads!), and I was set and ready for bed.

As soon as I got it out, I called my daughter Trinity to tell my renter it was out because she was getting worried about that now, since it was taking like 45 minutes, not a long time to me but to orthodox medicine it's an eternity! I was worried she'd call 911. Well, she did call the hospital her daughter is a nurse at…but luckily she told them not to come and they respected it. That was a close one! I would have been so freaking annoyed! She made up for it by feeding me and my kids.

All was well and it was done! Seven days past due, 11 lbs of baby boy was out plus placenta. The kids went to school, placenta was frozen for consuming later, Mommy, Willow and Yacu slept and relaxed all day. My darling niece, an Emergency Room doctor, came to visit a few days later, and I had her do the honors of weighing him. She also gave me an ultrasound a few weeks before the birth and I had the placenta placement confirmed. It was nice to know where to feel for it.

A Wild Ride
Submitted by Amy Bauman

IT WAS THE BEST of times, it was the worst of times…Oh wait, that's already been used.

Crosby's story is unique. Just a forewarning, if you know me in real life, if you are my husband's friend, if you are family, maybe even if you know me from church…You MAY want to turn back now! I mean it. TURN BACK NOW. Unless you want to know me…Unless birth is a normal/good thing to you…You may want to second guess not skipping this one. Things are about to get real here. We are about to enter into a relationship of TMI because BIRTH. That's right, BIRTH, and it's all a messy little beautiful wild crazy ride.

Crosby's story was a wild ride straight from the start. I was going through a range of emotions, I'd had a tough year. Just been through some things (just like birth is messy, life can be messy too. Doesn't make it not beautiful folks. Just makes it a bit more interesting). I think I knew going into his birth it was going to be different (they are ALL different but I mean different different. Not bad different, just different). It began with excitement (heck it ended with excitement), but I wasn't sure where I wanted to birth.

I knew I didn't necessarily want to go through this experience alone, and I knew I wanted female support. Not necessarily for the birth, but possibly. I knew without a doubt I wanted it for the pregnancy. I began seeing a new midwife at my old office (I mean the office I went to for prenatal care with my others). Immediately, I loved her. We clicked. And she treated me like an intelligent human being (which gets you a big gold star in my book). She was smart. She did say a few fearful things that made me want to yell, "Um, that's not true, and I can't believe you believe that!" but in the grand scheme of things that is pretty par for the course.

I was even considering birthing at the birthing center, which (after we moved to a new town and bought our first house) meant it would be a drive. An hour and a half-ish drive. I still wasn't certain I wanted to birth outside of our home (something I take very seriously), but at least my options were open. I had options. We spoke openly about that.

I asked if there were any reasons they wouldn't accept me at the birth center. I kind of assumed they wouldn't based on my birthing history and was pleasantly surprised when she assured me that would be of no issue. My history looked great. This birth would totally be straight forward, and I have the bonus of a "proven pelvis."

Fast forward to the end of my pregnancy, and I arrived at one of my later prenatal appointments only to be asked, "So, we are going for a hospital birth right?" Ummmm…no! And that's when she laid it on me. The birth center would not in fact be open before my due time (which was soon), although I had been led to believe it would the entire pregnancy. At the last appointment I was still being told, "Oh, definitely it will be!" (Giant smile…I guess I never did look to see if her fingers were crossed.)

And then she continued on, saying something along the lines of even if it were I definitely didn't qualify to birth there. Too risky. Thanks for asking. My geriatric uterus might implode. I may bleed to death. I might need a hysterectomy, and with my age if bleeding does happen, how will they do the hysterectomy without me at the hospital? My only question was when did the first step to stopping bleeding become a full on hysterectomy…I mean, might we be jumping the gun, there? Could we perhaps just try avoiding the bleeding to begin with or stop it if it does happen? Spoiler alert: you can do that! I don't know…maybe that's too far fetched when you are as old, ragged, and worn down as this 33 year old!

They had apparently suddenly been told that they weren't going to be helping women at the birth center who had birthed 6 or more children. (What a coincidence, I'm a woman and I've had 6 babies previously.)

"You understand, right? You get why we can't. A hospital birth will be just fine, right?"

Ummmm...I'd rather not unless needed. And the kicker....she was moving. So even if I didn't get my birth center birth, and even if I was okay with birthing at the hospital after not birthing there since baby number three, even if even if even if...this midwife (who I had kind of grown to love) wouldn't be there anyway.

"But of course the other midwife is taking all my clients. You understand, right?"

To say I was devastated was an understatement. Even more, I was kind of angry. It felt like I had been strung along the whole time. Maybe I wasn't. Maybe she didn't know she was moving. Maybe she didn't know any of the other surprises she just unleashed on me...maybe she didn't always think I was just an aged walking uterus waiting to implode....maybe. But I had been open and honest on my end. I was very honest about my previous planned home births and very honest about the fact that I was really considering, almost leaning towards birthing out of my home this time. None of this decision had to do with safety, but I really was looking for the womanly support this time. I had my reasons.

So that was the day it became clear. VERY CLEAR. After having prayed for God to make it clear, it was very clear. (Thanks God!) I would once again be planning a home birth. Good thing I had been taking care of myself like I was planning a home birth anyway. So plans changed. I honestly grew to more than just accepting them but being excited about them.

Fast forward, closer to the time Crosby was born. It was Labor Day morning. I woke up (early for me) around 8 a.m. and contractions started. I got up to shuffle around the house in the quietness as everyone else was asleep. I got on Facebook and chatted with a friend or two. Told them today might be the day. *Might* being the key word. (I maybe had said this a few times before). I told them about the contractions I'd been having pretty much consistently since 8. We laughed and chatted about clown cars…or fingertips…I can't remember the inside joke we had going here, but it was really funny.

I sat in the kitchen, music blaring, probably Skillet. I had been listening to the song "Lions" kind of on repeat the past few days. It's kind of an excellent birth anthem and really a life anthem (I dare you to look it up!). I spent a bunch of time screwing hardware back on our newly painted kitchen cabinets. Did I mention we decided to start redoing our kitchen the day Crosby was due? Can I just say I totally recommend it! Definitely helps in the patience department. Don't worry, we still haven't finished it. Raise your hand if you know how after baby comes everything else in your life pales and you don't care anymore!

At around noon I told my husband, "I'm pretty sure SURE today is the day." I think he believed me, maybe. Contractions were still nothing to write home about, but they were still there for sure. It was exciting.

Around 1:30 we decided we would walk the couple of blocks from our house to the local Labor Day Parade (just Austen and me). Kalel was given the big brother job of babysitting, and we told him we were going on a walk and would be back soon. He liked that. Our kids like being at home so they were totally happy about it.

As we walked, I think I told Austin a thousand times that "I feel really bad that our kids aren't coming. We really should be taking them to the parade." He assured me that seeing as I was in labor it was okay if they didn't get to come just this once. I laugh now at my obsession with this. I really felt like a terrible mother in the moment (well, sort of terrible, I still did it! Ha.) We walked along the sidewalks among the crowd getting ready for the parade. We definitely had to stop, and OFTEN. Things were getting way more intense. (Yay for walking! this is EXACTLY what we were hoping for.)

We joked and laughed a lot. I felt a bit awkward because I would be walking and then BAM! have to stop right then and there because of a big one. And then trying to keep a smile on my face and talk nonchalantly while in labor was fun too. Or stopping quickly in the middle of the sidewalk and then realizing someone was walking right behind us. Oops! When I say they got intense, I mean intense.

At one point I remember telling Austin, "These people wanna see a parade? I'll show them a parade!" It was great.

As we rounded our last corner, I was feeling like I'd rather get down on hands and knees, but if I did I may or may not get back up, so I didn't. We stopped to chat during a contraction, and I remember thinking, "I am so glad we don't know people very well yet. I can't imagine having to stop and talk to people right now."

Also, at one point he was pointing out a truck he liked parked in a random driveway and he was going on and on and on…and I remember thinking, "That's great…but please shut up. I am trying to be in horrible pain here. Can you just shhhhh…" Of course, I just nodded like I could feign interest and tried not to die. He did the same thing when we walked by a trailer for hauling things. He started telling me all about his plans for our trailer, and how he would paint it and I almost smacked him in the face. (But if I had I would have smacked him with a smile so that gets me a gold star right?)

I think I told him then, "Okay we need to get home now or you'll be carrying me home!" Not that that made it so we could move any faster, but still. It helped my brain just to say it. I think the last few blocks were full of my saying, "I'm gonna die. I'm gonna die. I'm gonna die." A twisted mantra if you will. (To clarify I knew I wasn't going to actually die. I was just being overly dramatic and a big baby because it hurt. Birth hurts. Yep. In case you forgot or haven't experienced it yet. Still worth it!)

Finally, we made it back home. I started a bath. After three hospital "land" births and three home water births, for some reason (a very stupid one!) I had thought, "Hmmm…I don't need a pool. Heck, maybe I'll even birth on land this time. Who knows. I think every time I tried to imagine it, I was upstairs in our bed delivering. I still held out hope I might use our clawfoot tub, and didn't order a new pool, so it was either the tub or nothing.

I soaked in the tub a bit and started to feel pushy. I had the radio on in there and the lady on the station said something about, "You know what the great thing about Labor Day is? Almost NO ONE has to labor!" I got a good chuckle out of that one. Did I mention the water had taken away a lot of the pain? I could laugh again….and then it started getting uncomfortable again, and I just couldn't get the full range of motion I needed to relax myself in the tub. Or, let's just face it, to cope at all. (This is when I could have used my beloved fishy pools of the past.) So I moved upstairs. Probably sprinted up the stairs because I knew once I got going and once I was out of the water there would be a BIG ONE. If I didn't get there in a straight shot I would be miserable and on the stairs.

I do not know what time it was or how much time I spent upstairs. It was not a comfortable time. YOWEEEE! Austin came in and out and mostly I kept asking him to leave. (Sorry husband. I really do love you.) I just needed to be alone.

I should say here I had him check the heartbeat a few times during all of this; that morning, before we went on our walk, when we got home, you know whenever I needed that reassurance. With our other home births I had always done that part using my stethoscope or fetoscope. There is something exhilarating about checking on your baby yourself. But during this baby we had discovered that if Austin laid his ear on my belly he could hear it and count and tell me what it was and that was just kind of our special thing this pregnancy. It really was sweet and cute and just a neat thing. So I had him check ear-to-belly again.

There is just something about that connection. It's a pleasant memory. And in the times of "I can't do this anymore!" it really helped me to know baby was doing just fine. NOTHING was wrong. WE. COULD. DO. THIS. Did I mention how super cute it was doing that ear to belly? It gives me the warm fuzzies just to remember it. Who knew even 7th babies get their own "special thing." So sweet.

So, this seems to be about the time I started SCREAMING! Normally, I'm a rather quiet, peaceful, internal birther. NOT THIS TIME. When I say screaming, I mean SCREAMING. I grew up across from the old meat locker in my town. When they brought hogs in to butcher them…YEAH THAT'S WHAT I SOUNDED LIKE! (I'm sure it was fun for all within ear shot.) I did have the kids giggling. I could hear them outside the door. That's when I would yell GO AWAY! And then Austin would come save me from them and their giggling and tell them to go back downstairs. Glad I could be amusing for them, but in the moment their giggling was not amusing for me. I do remember thinking, "Okay don't yell. you'll be able to relax more if you don't yell." and then a contraction would come, and I might get through one, but eventually there I was yelling again. I thought to myself "Screw it! And who says I can't yell anyway! I'm the boss here and I'm in pain! I am about as relaxed as I'm going to be" (ie: not at all).

So I went through a gajillion more contractions upstairs on our bed. I transitioned from all fours, on my back, back to all fours with head on a pile of pillows, semi squat, and back to on my side or flat on my back again. I yelled, yelled, and yelled some more. When I finally found my composure, then I had enough sense to yell again. I'm sure I was super fun to be around. Around this time Austin was back in the room for good and telling me he needed to call his work again to make sure they got his message that he wouldn't be in tonight for work. UM, NO!

I could not let him go do that and I was not hesitant to tell him he would not be leaving my side. He said it would only take a second. Yeah, he didn't win that one, and it soon became clear I wouldn't be letting him leave. I had been pushing off and on from the time I had come upstairs. (I started pushing off and on in the bathtub actually.) I was pushing with all my gumption for as long as felt instinctively right and safe and it just felt like baby wasn't moving. (Moving down I mean.) It was just hard. Hard. Hard. Hard. And I've had six babies. This was by far the hardest for me, and the most difficulty I've had coping with the pain.

In hindsight I really think it was all mental. This block. I don't really want to explain why, but just know if you are going through anything or have things in your life you haven't dealt with mentally, it truly can affect your delivery. Bonus advice: work through any fears you might have as well as any unresolved tension in your life before it's time for your baby to be born. Your body and your brain will thank you for it.

It got to the point where I said to Austin, "You know I don't take this decision lightly but I REALLY think we need to go in." (To the hospital, I meant.) In between contractions we talked about this as much as I could. There wasn't a big break but I tried to convey my message to him quickly and clearly before another one would hit. He understood, and after much talking we decided yes, we would go in. Let me clarify, nothing was wrong. Nothing was wrong with me. Nothing was wrong with baby. I just had this overwhelming feeling of, "We should probably go in now."

So Austin quickly got dressed. (When I say quickly I mean in labor land it took him about 7 and a half hours, it was probably less than a minute.) It's good to not look like a hobo when you transfer from a home birth to a hospital birth. He went down and talked to the kids and told them what was happening. When he came back up he was like, "Are you sure you want to go in? Why don't you have clothes on yet?" (…are you kidding me???) Followed quickly by, "Oh do you want me to bring you some pants?" And then it became clear he would be dressing me also. So he kept trying to, and I kept not letting him. I kept saying, "Just a minute. After this one." And I was praying. And I was still in lots of pain because birth. (I do not want to downplay how much pain I was in at this moment.)

Finally, he got them on me, leggings of course, and waited for me to attempt to get up off the bed. But every time I even thought about moving, another one would come. I kept saying, "Just a minute. After the next one." I think secretly he may have been laughing at me at this point, but he wasn't letting it show. I started imagining him carrying me downstairs because I didn't much feel like walking. (I think I even imagined him throwing me over his shoulders like a sack of potatoes. Ha.) Then I was imagining how I would end up just getting out the car and giving birth right in front of our young, single, male neighbor with my butt hanging halfway out the car and I thought, Hmmm…maybe this isn't such a good idea.

That's when I started praying more. And pushing more. And being in pain more. (Okay it was really the same but at the end of labor it can seem like more. That's how you know you're almost dead…er… I mean there!) So, I finally whispered/yelled to myself, "I can do this!" That's when Austin said he KNEW without a doubt we were staying home. I like that about him. He knows me too well. Sometimes you just have to be your own biggest cheerleader! You are the only you who can do this!

I began pushing with earnest. I realized the baby was coming, and my pants were still on. I struggled for a while trying to pull them down, and Austin came to my rescue and helped me. I pushed some more and finally finally could feel what felt like crowning. I can't remember if I told Austin the baby was right there or not. I pushed and was up in sort of a backwards semi-squat on the bed. I felt that familiar ring of fire, and out came the head…Oh wait…it just felt like a head…then it burst! It was such a shock! It was the water bag. It came out like a giant balloon and then burst EVERYWHERE! It was the craziest feeling ever. Normally I am in the water when this happens and don't even notice it. Then I was like, "Aw crap! Seriously?!" I thought I was in the homestretch and done here. And then it hit me there would be more pain and who knows how many more contractions because his head was not RIGHT there.

I move all around as best I can, while feeling like I can't move, and I'm in pain. I decided to check myself, and I felt hair…HAIR! I said very loudly, "Oh, he has hair! He's right there and HE. HAS. HAIR." FINALLY. So I pushed and pushed and pushed, and he crowned FOREVER and twelve and a half days. Seriously, felt like forever, and finally I flipped to hands and knees. I kept pushing, and he was kind of sticky so I was shimmying, but it wasn't working. (It was really just not fast enough for my brain because sometimes that's how brains work. Brains can be hard to deal with during birth.)

Austin said, "Oh, his head, it's huge!" and I said or thought, "I know. I felt it!" He said, "He's kind of blue." and I said back with a chuckle, "That's okay. Blue's good. White is bad." Just means he is getting blood and oxygenation. That's a good thing. I kept pushing little by little. Then Austin put his hand on my thigh (he said he thought that would help and it really did), and pushed just a tiny bit on my inner thigh with his hand. That was enough to release him and give him enough room to jiggle out more.

And then I swear I had to push for his belly and his butt to come out more. I sort of laid his head down on the bed after squatting my back legs down a little, and then birthed the rest of him, if that makes sense. So I both birthed and caught him and set him down gently all in one drawn-out fell swoop. Then I leaned back and picked him up and he let out a cry for us, kind of a wail. (I forgot to mention that when he was sort of born but only his head was out he let out the cutest little whimper. Sort of sounded like a little baby cat. It was the cutest, most wonderful little noise ever. And it sure gave me that little oomph to go on so I could get down to meeting him.)

After that we loved him, and I immediately said, "Go get the kids! Go get the kids!" Did I mention this was our first daytime-only labor and birth?! Crazy how new things happen each and every time, even with your seventh baby. He really was lucky baby number seven! We love him so much, and I so hope his story was worth the wait because he was so worth all of it, the whole thing!

May this story of a hard birth, of pain, of uncertainty even be inspiring. May it be an encouragement that even in the hard times, good things happen. New life is worth it no matter how it comes. Family is our greatest gift (apart from Jesus of course…well, WITH Him I suppose!) trials and all. This, my friends, is why I'm a birth nerd, and now I can't wait to have another…

Oops! Did I just say that out loud?

Tranden Excalibur's Unassisted Birth
Submitted by Amy Bauman

IN HONOR OF THE new year, I decided to get to it and type up the birth of Tranden Excalibur. When praying about how to go about posting this, I was perplexed as to how to start off. I do not want to offend, nor do I feel like I should apologize. I know unassisted birth is a touchy subject and birth itself is very personal. I thought about posting the reasons we chose this route but feel that might detract from the story itself…and after all this is Tranden's story, not mine.

I will just start off by saying birth is very near to my heart, and it's something I take seriously. This took months of planning. Years, really. It wasn't something we stepped into lightly. If you are someone who has made different birthing/pregnancy choices, I think that is completely wonderful. I think mammas who make informed decisions, whatever they be, are great! And just as I respect your choices, I hope that you will show us that same encouragement.

On the morning before Tranden's actual birthday I woke up pregnant, yet again! Being just as convinced as I was the day before that I was clearly in labor, I rolled over and begged my husband to stay home from work. We both laid there talking about our hesitancy in keeping him home another day. After much listing of pros and cons it was clear he would yet again being staying home.

Labor was on! Problem was, the contractions weren't so much. I can honestly say I just knew. I knew I needed my partner, Austin, there for mental support as well as to wrangle the kids so I could concentrate on letting my body relax and do what it needed to do. Having been 5 centimeters dilated for about three weeks now, people tend to doubt that the real deal will ever actually conspire. I, on the other hand, was hopeful. I know my body works! I know it is an intricate process! I know it takes time!

Did I get impatient at times? Yes. Did I ever consider throwing in the towel and going to the hospital and letting them break my water or a number of things that would have been done when they realized how far dilated I was and that I had been laboring on and off for quite some time? Yes! It was one of those times where you just want to meet your baby soooooo bad (in our case, just want to know if babe is a girl or a boy...although I was CERTAIN he was a girl... yes, I said he!) I decided we would do the next best thing: enjoy our final day as a family of 5! I was a little concerned Austin would get in trouble staying home, and that his boss would think he was playing hooky. I mean, it's pretty hard to tell your boss, "Yes, my wife was 5 cm dilated and yes we were at the park and yes she is in labor but no she isn't in pain." For some reason, because of our fast food/birth mentality I don't think he would have bought it...and even if he had that would be just one more person telling us to go in and "let them help us start things moving."

Nah, we prefer to fly under the radar. I had already skipped my last doctors appointment, knowing I was dilated a lot and knowing there is no way they would be happy with me going home to let labor take its course. So we woke up, got dressed, and had breakfast. I made my "death tea"...Austin's nice name for my red raspberry leaf tea. I asked if he wanted a sip, he said he wouldn't drink it EVER! We then proceeded to go to the park and to the library, where I read Frankie a book 6 million times with something in the title about mommy having a baby...this is a book she had become very attached to every single library visit for the past six weeks or so. The boys played video games, and Austin and I talked, mostly about the coming child and what would happen if I really wasn't in labor and he had to go to work on Monday with no baby news.

He kept track of the rambunctious group while I took a quick trip to see my favorite Chiropractor. She adjusted me, we laughed about how I was sure the week before that I wouldn't be in again. We joked about this getting me all lined up for baby to shoot right out!

Then I set up my next appointment and said, as always, "I hope I don't see you next week."

I stopped by Grand Central and picked up supplies for Labor Day Cookies. (I have since found out these are the basic same ingredients that women have used for quite sometime in the "groaning cake" generally baked during early labor.) After getting all of the ingredients that I didn't have at home, I swung by the library and picked up the rest of the clan, and we headed home. I baked cookies. "Death cookies," they were later named...notice a theme here? They did taste and smell awful. I ate as many as I could handle (3) and decided that was it, I was taking a nap and labor would pick up. So Austin took the boys and Frankie outside to play basketball, swing, burn off energy, and, most importantly, leave mama alone! Mama may have been a little teensy bit grumpy! I laid down and proceeded to nap and woke up about two hours later DEFINITELY IN LABOR!

These contractions were different. They almost followed a scale. They would start suddenly, intensify slowly, and then work back to nothing. I KNEW THIS WAS IT! I smiled, almost scared, thinking surely if I knew I was in labor it would somehow stop the whole thing. This is three days after my EDD, by the way. I went to the bathroom, made some more death tea, and happily walked outside. I'm pretty sure there was a skip in my step now. Oh yeah, I also realized I was 6 cm now (that was back up in the bathroom, by the way.) So, I walk out the door and wave to my husband who is too caught up in impressing the 8 year olds with his half-court shot. I say, "Austin! Austin!" and I smile and give him a thumbs up. We chat and decide it's time for a walk. The boys wail, knowing they have to walk, no bikes this time. Frankie gets excited and we head out.

Upon walking our usual route Frankie gets super excited and runs and trips over her own feet and falls and bonks her head. A real nice goose egg! On the bright side, she happily fell asleep in my arms and snoozed the rest of the way home. We returned home and daddy filled the birth pool with the help of two little excited boys. They settled in to watching Scooby Doo on the T.V. in our room, sprawling across the bed. I spent time in Frankie's room (you know, the one she doesn't sleep in but happens to have pink curtains?!)

I leaned on the birth ball just enjoying myself. We posed for some pictures, courtesy of our little photographer Kalel. Eventually, the kids fell asleep and the contractions got stronger. I decided I would get in the water and relax. I spent some time in there and Frankie woke up and joined me. She had fun splashing, "swimming", and rubbing my back. She got tired and made her way to the family bed and fell asleep too. That is when it really picked up.

Austin helped with hip pressure as Tranden was moving down, as well as counter pressure on my back. Eventually, I said, "Okay, that's enough, you can leave me alone now, nothing is really helping now." And that he did. He watched a little news radio and I labored on. I only freaked out on him once. He entered the room, and I yelled, "Ew, gross! You brushed your teeth didn't you?" My pregnant senses were on overload and that did not please me. I proceeded to apologize immediately following the contraction. He also fixed the lamp on the nightstand beside the pool, and I yelled at him for that too. Which I also apologized for one second later.

Eventually we came to pushing. I began doing grunty pushing at the end of every other contraction. It felt great, like I was actually doing something, and it took the edge off a little. At first, I worried in my mind about "What if I am pushing too soon?" But that was quickly wiped away by, "Well, I couldn't stop pushing even if I wanted to."

I pushed off and on for almost three hours. It was great, powerful, scary, everything. I wish I had said out loud some of the thoughts going through my head at the time. On video they would have been very funny. My husband took care of the obvious while I labored on. He basically left me alone (not physically, he was in the room), and that was the best thing he could have done at the time. It's what I needed. I had little conversations in my head about "How can I get to the hospital and get them to give me an emergency c-section?" But then I freaked out thinking, "They won't give me one, there is no medical reason. I have to make them think there is a reason. Well, that won't work, they will be so mad at me for trying to do this at home that they will take their time helping me and really make me wait it out."

Then I was thinking, "Man, now I see why women get the epidural!" Then I was freaking out thinking, "What if I'm not even dilated, and I'm pushing and in pain for nothing?" I quickly reminded myself, "Duh, you already checked and are fully dilated. You can feel the head right there, you're just going to have to do it." Yes, I midwifed myself.

It was as if in that moment a lightbulb went off, and there he was. I remember Austin being in the bathroom and I said, "Baby! baby!" To which he ran in and said, "He's right there!" So out came his head, and it was as if time was suspended with me thinking, Wow, that is a really cool whitish bag…the contraction was over, and I waited for another and then his shoulders were out, and about the time his stomach emerged the water bag burst.

It was cool. He was the cleanest baby I had ever seen! He came out crying and pink and flailing his arms. I brought him up and Austin said, "What is it? What is it?" To which I replied, "I don't care!" Then I looked, and sure enough, he was a boy!

Talk about shock! Yay! So we waited, and eventually I clamped and cut the cord. Then I got out and loved my baby! Within three minutes I was back leaning over the pool to deliver the placenta and the rest is history. Not much left as far as the story goes.

We loved our baby, I fed him, we weighed him, and he took a bath with me. We called a friend and had her stop by because we were just so excited! She got me juice and helped us settle back into bed for the night. She also took the coolest picture of us and you can see the three kids snoozing in the background. It was the greatest most undramatic birth ever.

Tranden Excalibur was born!

As a side note, Joaquin was the only one of the siblings to meet him before morning. He woke up an hour or so after the fact and walked in where we were holding Tranden before we returned to bed. He came in and looked at us. We excitedly announced, "Joaquin look! It's your new baby brother! Mommy had the baby!" He stared, said nothing, and turned and walked away. (I kind of assumed he was sleepwalking and wouldn't remember a thing.)

That was until the next morning I heard him proudly proclaiming to everyone, his brother, his sister, and later to kids on the playground, "I was the first one to see my baby brother after he was born! It was so cool!" Of course he had a huge smile plastered across his face that he couldn't have wiped off if he wanted to! The kids have been smitten ever since, as have Austin and I!

A Christmas Unassisted Birth
Submitted by Amy Bauman

TUCKER EVANGELIQUE

Oh, sweet Tucker, our happy girl! I don't even know how to start her story but I know without a doubt it needs to be told. I cannot quit thinking about it, can't even wash dishes without my mind transporting back to that day screaming, "Write this down, it needs to be shared! You don't know who you will inspire. Remember how much reading others stories has helped you? Remember how reading about how normal and everyday birth is helped you? How it helped you sort through your questions? Go and be that for someone else. I wrote this story, share it!"

Oh, how far I have come from being hugely pregnant with Kalel and hiding my copy of The Womanly Art of Breastfeeding, Spiritual Midwifery, and the 5 Safe Standards for Childbearing behind other boring books as I hand the librarian my quarters to pay for them at the Library book sale in nowhere Kansas. AHHH, WHAT IF SHE SEES WHAT I'M READING?!? Makes me chuckle.

Tucker's pregnancy started off like any other; the excitement, the appointments, but it was different. Between living in a new city, having less-than-encouraging ultrasounds, and our car accident, something just seemed different this time around. I couldn't put my finger on it. Spent lots of time seeking the Lord and being encouraged by Him. Contrary to popular belief, every birth IS different. They individually deserve care and consideration as to making plans as to where and with whom (or without) you should give birth. Really, like everything else, it just takes time to think it through, to wait for answers, and to listen, to listen and wait again.

It wasn't until a week before she was born when I finally felt the green light: this will be another family-only home birth. It was such a quiet, exciting time. Fast forward to Christmas Eve. It was a slow, lazy day. It would be the first Christmas Season we would NOT spend with my husband's family and only the second Christmas he could ever remember not being at his grandma's house. Tucker had bigger plans for us! We were kind of in a mopey "we should be there, not here" mood. Excited at the possibility of a new baby joining us but not convinced she was really coming, we decided to go out to do some last minute shopping and eat at our favorite pizza place.

We had a conversation on the way there about how we really could just leave now and make it in time for the festivities at his grandma's house. We could surprise everyone. And we knew our kids would be so happy. We talked about how we obviously wouldn't have a baby today anyway, so it really wouldn't matter. But something kept us home anyhow, which is far from normal for us.

We decided to eat first then head to the store. I really needed to get to the store and purchase some newborn diapers, pads, and I wanted to pick up some stocking stuffers with a little extra money we happened to have. We have never filled their stockings so we thought that would make it a little more special. When we got to the restaurant and filled our plates (after giving our boys our usual pep-talk about eating their money's worth, i.e., eat lots!) I noticed some minor tightenings. Stronger than usual but no pain really. I got a little bit excited.

When I finished eating, I decided to use the restroom and do a little bit of checking just to see. (I swear I planned to not eat any more or touch ANYTHING I swear). So Frankie and I went to the ladies room (Am I the only one to ever check herself at the local pizza joint?!). I said to her, do you realize this could be the last time we ever eat here before the baby is born? This could be our last time as a family of six going anywhere! Of course we smiled like goons and giggled. She went in one stall and I in the other and whoa, baby, was I surprised, we are talking major dilation, and something I had never felt before, the bag bulging like crazy.

I was almost in shock. Happily of course! We washed up (super extra well). We returned to our table, I'm sure I was the freak who couldn't wipe the smile off her face for anything. I leaned over to my husband and said, "Two words: Bulging. Bag." of course he looks at me frightened and says, "Gross." Then he says, "I don't really know what that means, but do we need to go?" I had to inform him it did not mean the baby was hanging out of me, but we probably should hurry and try and get home unless we want clean up by the buffet. That's when he decided we really couldn't leave until he had a few more cinnamon rolls. I made the mistake of eating one off his plate and I quickly learned that was unacceptable, even in my having a baby state! We finally loaded up, and when I say finally, you must realize it takes us FOREVER to do anything!

We still have to head to Walmart, but I am in power-shop mode. We have things to do and I still have to wrap presents! We do our shopping, chuckling that we are the only people to wait till baby's due date to go buy the necessities. (I did that on purpose so I would have something to do in labor. Bonus points for me!) I finally say as we are shopping, "Um we really REALLY need to go." So we get home and things settle down a little. We watch a family movie and get the kids asleep, making sure to tell them before they are out that we will probably have a new baby brother or sister in the morning, and ask if they would like to be woken up.

"YES!" they screech.

Finally, it's just Austin and I. We decide to watch "Music and Lyrics" (I think we have watched every funny movie we own in the last 3 days). After it's over I'm a bit discouraged. Nothing is really happening. I mean I'm still tightening but they aren't painful and they seem to have spaced out. I say, maybe we should just go to bed and if they pick up we will know it's the real deal, but I am out of hope. This was another false alarm.

Austins says, "I think we should just stay up. Let's watch another movie and see what happens." I say "Okay, then, well I guess you better fill the pool because I'm sure when it finally is time we won't have much time to fill it and I want it piping hot so I can use it when

I need it." I head off, discouraged, knowing nothing is happening anymore, sad that I thought this was it and just really really disappointed. I'm not prepared for this. When I got to wipe there is blood. BLOODY SHOW! (Only a pregnant woman could understand my new found enthusiasm) and almost like that here come the contractions again.

And boy are they intense! I go to Austin and proclaim, "This is it! It really is!" and spill way to many details. As always the response is, "Gross! Did you have to tell me that?" Happily I nod. He continues filling the pool. I remember going back to the bathroom and alternating between toilet and hands on knees with my head on the cold tile floor. Thank goodness I've super cleaned! And, oh thank the Good LORD I'm not at the hospital because I would not stick my face on that floor. Ick. I'm telling you it felt so good!

When I return to the living room the tub is filled. Warm bath, I love thee. The living room is beautiful with only the light of the Christmas tree right by the pool. Just how I'd imagined. Kids are sleeping. Just Austin and I and the quiet of the night. It seems right after I get in I'm in great pain. "Oh what was I thinking?!" I alternated between the tub and the bathroom on hands and knees, enjoying the cool floor. Cold. HOT. Cold. HOT. Back in the tub I'm leaning over the side feeling the urge to push and thinking "This is way too early! But then…I don't know what else to do!"

So I would gruntily push and then sit back and sleep, push, sit back and sleep. That's when I'm thinking, while pushing, "OH, this is why women get the epidural. How long will it take us to load up, get to a hospital, and get hooked up? No, no that would be torture, the ride there, in the car with no tub, noooo!" Then I'm thinking, "Oh, next time I am having my baby at the hospital and I'm getting drugs, that's just the way it is." And then, "Oh, no next time I'm having surgery. I'm just setting it up. Right from the beginning. I'll set up the date and explain it later. Oh oh no this is it! I'm not having more kids. I'm not. I'm just not. I cannot do this again. I won't!" And then I chuckle thinking, "Yeah, after this baby is out you'll be begging for another. You will," and I smile.

Well, I decide, I just have to get through this, and whining isn't helping, so get over yourself and quit being a baby. I begin pushing every other contraction. I lean over and ask Austin, "Do you think it's too soon to push?" and he says, "If your body is telling you to then I'd say it knows what's going on better than I." Perfect words. I love my husband! He then leaves to get something and comes back, and I hear music starting. He had picked out a CD from our old collection when we were first married and put it into the player. The words start, "It'd be much easier if only I could see you. If only I had a face to put with the name I love..." I have never even thought of having this music in my playlist which I now can't use because our computer is being stupid, but it's perfect. And with those words, these songs, suddenly I can do it. I'm having a baby!

Immediately, suddenly, right then... yes, I am being redundant but it went from not there to there! Bam!

The clouds open, the heavens parted, and whoa baby, there is a baby right there. I KNOW the next push is it! I KNOW it. I say, "Austin, Austin, Baby, the baby is coming!" and sit back on my ankles and push with all my might. Nothing happens. I can feel he or she is stuck. Not scary, the sky is falling, dangerous stuck, just plain you need to move stuck. Her head is out but the rest of her isn't moving yet, and my brain says "You are going to have to change positions a few times so babe can spiral out." So I do. Hands and knees, squatting, leaning forward, and POP! Out flies the body. I catch her and bring her up, saying, "Oh we have a baby! We have a baby! Look at all that hair! How does OUR BABY have ALL THAT HAIR?!"

I say, "wake up the kids, wake up the kids." While Austin is trying to rouse the sleeping bears I think, "I should wait to check who he/she is, no I can't. Oh well."

"It's a girl! It's a girl! Tucker Evangelique! It's Tucker!" Kalel flies off the couch where he was sleeping by the pool. He is awake, the boy who you can't rouse unless you can muster up an earthquake is off the couch leaning over the pool saying, "Oh she's so cute! Can I hold her? Can I hold her?" (It was ADORABLE!) He was smitten. I tell him, let's wait just a minute. Let me get her unconnected first.

That was apparently an okay answer, but he stared at her like she was the only person in the universe, and he was wearing one of those smiles you can't hide even if you want to. We cut the cord, and

Austin helped him hold her on the couch while I moved to the recliner to get the placenta out. (It was covered in chux pads and blankets, don't worry.) Boy, those after pains were a doozy. It was taking a bit longer and I was losing a bit more blood than I was comfortable with, so I did end up putting a bit of the membranes from near the cord in my cheek. Just pulled off and whopped it in when Austin wasn't looking, lest he gag. Pretty quickly the blood slowed and out plopped the placenta. Ahhh…much better.

After that I cuddled my baby, bathed with her, moved to the bed, and wrapped stocking stuffers. It was four in the morning, and I had nothing to do but gaze at my little baby and take her all in. Oh, and wrap presents! It was a good day, an amazing Christmas morning, a joyous day to add a new member to our family!

Tucker Evangelique, our little Christmas baby was born bright and early and by the tree. It was the best Christmas ever! I couldn't get on the phone fast enough to call and tell people the good news!

Short and Sweet
Submitted by Sarah

I WAS 41 WEEKS 4 days, and knew that the pregnancy journey for my fourth child would come to a close soon. Would this be the birth I had always wanted? I spent the day as I spent any other day on the farm: milked the goats, came inside, and drew a bath. I had a feeling today would be the day.

During the bath, I had my first contraction. I knew immediately that this was labor. Because it was early labor (so I thought), I thought I'd relieve myself to get the system moving.

I had planned to birth in the barn, but this crisp February day and the length of the labor wouldn't allow that. Two more contractions and my perfect daughter was born en caul into my arms.

While labor was intense, it also was somewhat pleasurable, and gave me such a wave of empowerment.

The Freebirth of Eliza May
Submitted by Rosie Parton

ELIZA MAY

March 8, 2018

I wasn't due for another week and a half, and both of the boys had arrived on their due dates, so I was not expecting labor for at least another week. On Thursday the 2nd of August, I woke up to my waters leaking, and they leaked a lot all day long. I was a little bit concerned because we were moving house the next day, but I knew that it could still be days or even weeks away, and I was confident that Bubba would wait until we were settled. That night I got some very strong contractions. Okay, so maybe it was going to happen soon.

Throughout Thursday night I was woken by about 7 or 8 very strong contractions that I needed to breathe and focus through. I knew these were labor contractions and not just Braxton Hicks.

On Friday morning, the removalists showed up at 7 a.m. Dan went to work, and the contractions pretty well stopped. I only had 4 or 5 all morning; my body knew I couldn't birth with these people around. The boys and I went to the house with the removalists with their first load so I could tell them where to put everything. I had two contractions on the way there that were very intense, and in hindsight I wonder if I should have been driving…

After they unloaded the truck and left, and it was just the boys and me at the house, the contractions picked up straight away to about 5 minutes apart lasting about a minute and very intense. I asked my sister-in-law to come over and play with the boys so I could do some unpacking, and I called Dan to come home from work. By the time he got home contractions were about 2-3 minutes apart.

A bit of a back story is needed here: in December 2017, six days after we found out I was pregnant, two 35-meter trees fell on/through our roof during a freak storm. We had been in temporary accommodation ever since while insurance repaired our home.

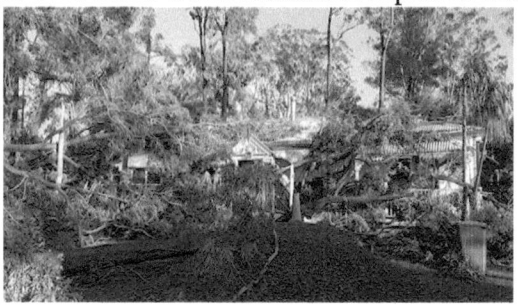

Damage from the storm

It was the most stressful, strange, difficult eight months of my life, but we were finally moving home just in time for the baby to arrive. We thought it would happen once we were maybe a little bit more settled in.

During my pregnancy, I had horrific pain in my groin and leg from varicose veins. I had it during my previous pregnancies, though far less severe, and I had gone through 3 surgeries to fix the issue, but they hadn't worked, as I found out about 7 weeks into pregnancy. Despite wearing a compression brace for my pelvis and full length compression stockings from the moment I got out of bed till the moment I went to bed every day, I couldn't stand up for more than about 10 minutes at a time or it became too painful. If I didn't wear the compression garments, about 1 minute was the limit.

As you can imagine, it was very difficult to remain optimistic; we were out of our home, I was in debilitating pain trying to be a good mum to my 2 and 4-year-old boys and trying to do the basics like washing, cooking and cleaning while not being able to stand up for pain. I was so thankful to a beautiful friend who came regularly to help me with washing and cooking, but it was still hard. Not to mention the countless hours of stress and paperwork and phone calls and research and emails that go with insurance claims. I think I was suffering depression; it was a huge struggle to get out of bed every day, knowing that I had a day of pain and stress ahead of me.

At 11 weeks I almost lost the baby. I started cramping, then bleeding, a lot. I held onto Dan and cried and cried and told him I didn't want to lose the baby. He just responded with, "I know," and held onto me. I laid down for a few hours and texted some dear friends, one of whom replied with photos of pages from the book "Supernatural Childbirth" with scriptures and prayers to declare in case of threatened miscarriage. I lay still, tears streamed down my face, and I whispered the prayers and declarations over and over and asked the baby to please stay in there and to please be okay. The next day I got an ultrasound. I am anti-ultrasounds, but in this case I believe that the stress of not knowing if my baby was alive or not would have done more damage than the ultrasound. I asked the sonographer if there was a heartbeat, and as soon as she replied, "Your baby is fine," I couldn't stop the tears of gratitude from flowing. I still had my baby.

At around 20 weeks I decided I wanted to freebirth, and Dan supported me 100%. I had been playing with the idea, but after reading and watching a lot of birth stories from women who had done it, I knew that's what I wanted too. Freebirthing is about taking birth from being a medical procedure, and returning it to being a normal, completely instinctive, natural process. I had beautiful, natural, midwife-attended home births for the first two, but looking back on those births, for me, having a medical professional present was an interference and hindrance in itself. She didn't do anything wrong at all. In fact, she was a brilliant midwife, and I would recommend her to anyone wanting a home birth.

I found that having a medical professional there made me doubt my own instinct, and I felt like I needed to run everything by her to make sure it was "okay." I wasn't in charge of my own birth. This time, I wanted my birth to be fully instinctual, fully un-medical and fully mine, the way it was designed to be and the way it was for centuries. I told my midwife I wanted to freebirth, and she was so supportive and gracious; she even checked over my research and lists to make sure I was fully prepared. I educated myself on what to do in any emergency situation, and I learned that situations that constitute a true emergency are extremely rare.

I knew I could transfer to hospital if one of those super rare emergencies did happen, and I knew beyond a doubt that my birth was far more likely to be easy and straightforward at home than at hospital. I knew I was giving myself and my baby the best chance of a calm, beautiful, natural birth; completely unhindered and completely instinctive. We decided not to tell many people at all because I knew that most wouldn't understand, and would try to talk me out of it. I was very excited.

We still didn't know when we would be moving home, so I couldn't do anything to prepare my "birth space" or do any nesting. I couldn't visualize the birth because I didn't know where it would be. I didn't even do much physical exercise or meditation and breathing practice like I did last time, simply because I didn't have time with everything we had going on, and I didn't have motivation because of how I was emotionally. In the month leading up to moving back home, Dan was camping at the house so he could work on it full time, so I was playing single mum and taking meals over to him once or twice a day. It was a mad rush to try and get everything (renovating, finishing things that insurance didn't do) done before we moved. We finally got the news from insurance that we would be moving home on the 3rd of August, just in time to move and get settled before the baby arrived. Or so we thought…

Halfway through moving day, just after Dan got home from work, we had to make a decision: stay at the house and just roll with whatever happened, or go to his parents' place to birth the baby. We both really wanted to birth at home, and besides, we still had the rest of the day of moving to get done, so we decided I would try lying down rather than pottering and unpacking to see if I could slow labor down.

It's important to understand the state of the house at this point. We were moving back into a completely empty, newly refurbished, but only partially completed, house. Dan had been converting our laundry room into a bathroom and our bathroom into an en-suite, but the en-suite wasn't even started yet and the bathroom was far from finished. It had our big bath in the corner, not even sealed yet. Some tiling was done, without the grout even cleaned off. Dan had literally done the grouting at midnight the night before. There was no vanity or bench or mirror or curtain or anything, and the washing machine was in the middle of the room. We were planning a water birth in the bath.

There was also nothing else in the house. Not a bed, not a sheet, not a towel. Everything was arriving dismantled or in boxes, and it was chaotic. I laid down in the swag that Dan had been camping in, and the contractions slowed right down to 10-15 minutes apart, but they were SO painful! I couldn't believe the difference.

It was agonizing laying there trying to sleep in between but waiting for and dreading the next inevitable excruciating contraction. It was so strange working against labor and trying to stop it from happening rather than working with the contractions as I had done last time. I realized that this must be what most women go through, simply because they are not educated on how to work with and surrender to the contractions, and they try to escape the pain. It was awful.

I stayed like that for the next 5 hours. It was the longest day of my life. Every time I got up to the go to the toilet, the contractions were straight back to 2 minutes apart, so I would rush back to the swag to ward them off again. My sister-in-law had to go, and my mother-in-law came and took over looking after the boys at 3 p.m. We had planned to have her at the house during the birth anyway to look after our 2-year-old.

As soon as the removalists brought our bed, Dan prioritized getting it assembled, and I moved onto the bed sometime in the afternoon. The removalists finally left at about 5:30 p.m. after chatting for AGES with Dan and taking their jolly time. They knew I was having contractions but didn't realise how far into labor I was. Dan didn't realize either, to be fair. I appeared calm most of the time, but the pain was so bad that I was struggling to stay in control. I called Dan into the bedroom just before they left and told him that laying down was starting to not work anymore, the contractions were getting closer together anyway. I had ordered Indian takeaway for dinner because I figured we would need to eat, and the delivery man showed up just after 5:30 p.m., and he also chatted to Dan for AGES. In my head I was screaming "JUST GO AWAY! I NEED TO GIVE BIRTH!"

As soon as the Indian man left, I got up out of bed and started walking through the house. The contractions were suddenly on top of each other with sometimes a minute in between, sometimes 10 seconds in between. Dan was putting sheets one the boys' beds so they could go to sleep, but I went and grabbed him and told him that it was going to be soon and that we needed to get things ready. We both started rushing around. The bath didn't even have a spout on it, so Dan was finding and attaching the spout, I was filling my water bottle and digging through boxes to try and find a bowl to birth the placenta into.

Dan watched me for a second and told me I was "transitioning." He could tell I was going into the zone. He frantically told me, "We haven't picked a boy's name!", and I told him it didn't matter. I went into the boys' bedroom and told Reuben that Bubba would be coming out soon. Dan's mum was putting Levi to bed, Dan was setting up the go-pro and I was getting out all the towels and a little chair for Reuben to sit on and the handheld mirror and a bucket...in-between contractions, of course. During contractions I was swaying, walking, and rotating my hips. I ended up swinging from the rafters on our back veranda to take the pressure off. I had never been this far into labor without being in water before, and I was surprised at how intense the pain was. While I was on the back veranda I got my first pushing contraction. I called out, "Hey Dan... I'm pushing."

He thought I was literally pushing the baby out right then and there. He asked what I wanted him to do, so I told him to fill the bath. I thought based on my previous births that I had about 15 minutes left, and I still wanted a water birth.

He started filling the bath. I went and got Reuben, then hopped in the ankle-deep water. It was cold. Dan flicked it to hot and it started warming up. I gave Reuben a pep talk, reminding him of all the birth videos we had watched, and that there would be blood and that it would probably hurt me, and reminding him to stay quiet. I had a pushing contraction, and Dan tried the hip squeeze that had been such a help in my last birth, but it was awkward because he wasn't in the bath, and it didn't really help anyway. Reuben loudly asked if we had remembered the scissors (he was very excited to cut the cord).

We reminded him to stay quiet. Dan changed the lightbulb from a fluoro to a soft white.

I had another pushing contraction, what was left of my waters broke, and then the water that was filling the bath started coming out yellow. We hadn't been living there for 8 months so the water had just been sitting in the pipes and had turned yellow. I asked Dan if that mattered for Bubba, and he confidently said it didn't, even though he didn't actually know. He knew I needed to stay calm and confident, and he knew I would be doubting whether I should stay in the bath if he gave me any reason to question it.

I asked Dan if the water was still getting warm. It wasn't. The hot water system had chosen that moment to die. So the water was tepid, it was yellow, and it was shallow, but there was no turning back now. Dan had caught the baby at the last birth, but because of the position I found myself in I told him I was going to catch it myself. I felt up inside me and I could feel the baby's head, only about an inch in. It was amazing. I could feel its hair, and I could actually feel the little tectonic plates of its head overlapping. Another contraction, then another rest. Dan rubbed my back. I said "No. Actually yes." I told Reuben he's a good boy. We all looked at the camera and smiled for a labor photo.

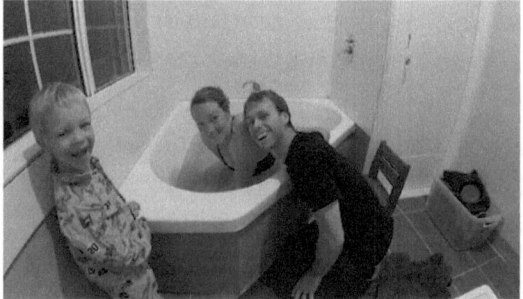

Another contraction. I knew it would be very soon. During this one, I suddenly had the irrational thought and feeling that the baby couldn't fit out. It didn't seem possible, and it was happening so fast that I had a moment of fear. I freaked out that I was going to tear. I told Dan I didn't want to tear, and he reminded me to just relax. Logically, I knew I wouldn't, but in that moment I was sure I just couldn't do it; it wasn't physically possible. The feeling passed with the contraction. Another brief break. I talked to the baby: "Hey Bubba, see you in a minute."

This was the first birth where I have been mentally present enough to even think of talking to the baby. The next contraction, I swore. I felt for a moment like a train with no breaks, like I had no control over what was happening and where I was going. To be honest, I felt like I was going to be torn apart. I didn't understand how the baby could fit through the birth canal and I felt stretched to my absolute limit. I deliberately and consciously submitted to the birthing process and trusted that my body knew what it was doing, even if my mind was having a bit of a flip-out. There was nothing I could do but let my body do what it needed to.

It turns out that was the final contraction. I had my hand on the baby's head as it emerged from me. It was so amazing. There was no "ring of fire", just a lot of pressure. As soon as the head was out there was so much relief but still so much pressure. I told Dan and Reuben, "Head's out," waited for a few seconds, then I felt the whole body rotate inside of me as it emerged all at once into the tepid, yellow water and its mama's waiting hands. It was 6:15 p.m., only 45 minutes after the removalists and delivery driver had left.

I scooped the baby up out of the water, exclaiming, "Oh my goodness, I just did it!" The baby started crying straight away, (probably because the water wasn't exactly a welcoming temperature!) Dan reached over and unwrapped the cord from the neck, and I held the little body against mine while I breathed out my relief and triumph and disbelief. I had done it. I had birthed my baby myself. It was such a wonderful, beautiful moment. I made a comment about the hair being brunette (after my two blondies, it was quite a surprise), then said "Hello Bubba, what are you?" Lifted and saw it's a girl!

It's a girl!

I had a feeling when I was pregnant that she was a girl, and while I would have been equally happy with another boy, my heart swelled with so much incomparable love when I realized I had a daughter. I was so overwhelmed that I cried and sobbed and then double checked. She was definitely a girl. A daughter. She had a big cake of vernix on her forehead, and she was totally perfect. We named her

Eliza May straight away. We had her name picked since before we even got married.

We sent Reuben to go get his little brother, and a very sleepy Levi came in and checked her out with a very happy grandma who had tears streaming down her face. She took Levi back to bed, and we let the yellow water out of the bath and wrapped ourselves up with towels. Eliza started breastfeeding straight away.

I went into a bit of shock and started shaking and shivering uncontrollably. I think it just happened so fast and it was so intense and it had been such a big, overwhelming day that I just couldn't process it all and my body reacted. I knew what to do though because I had educated myself. Dan wrapped me up in more towels and put a few drops of rescue remedy under my tongue, and I was fine within a few minutes. He helped me out of the bath and the placenta came easily within about 40 minutes. I took some homeopathic drops for the contraction pain and it seemed to help.

There was hardly any blood at all, and I hadn't torn or even grazed. I gave Eliza to Dan for some skin to skin while I got dressed, then we all headed to bed for more skin on skin and breastfeeding. After an hour or two, Dan tied the cord, and Reuben cut it with his craft scissors. Nothing was sterilized and everything was perfect.

Even though the birth was nothing like what I had imagined it would be, I had followed my instinct, I knew we were both safe every step of the way, and I never once wished I had a medical professional there. I was confident in my knowledge of birth and its variations, and in my innate ability to do what God designed me to do.

Reuben went to bed, Grandma went home, and Dan and I sat and reveled in the wonder of our new daughter and our amazing birth. We had done it; we had freebirthed our baby, in our home. I birthed and caught my own daughter, on my own terms, completely following my own instinct. It was the most amazing, empowering moment of my life. After everything we had been through in the last eight months, all of the pain, all of the stress, all of the trauma, she was our reward. She was the light at the end of our tunnel, our new beginning.

Dan told me how immensely proud of me he was, we relived every moment of the day, pinched ourselves because it all felt like a dream. We let our friends and family know she had arrived, weighed her on our kitchen scales, balancing on an esky lid, and measured her with my sewing tape. We were all tucked up ready to sleep by about 9:30 p.m., surrounded by unpacked boxes, chaos and peace.

Eliza May Parton 03/08/2018. 6:15 p.m. 7 lbs 2 oz, 19.6 inches. Freeborn at home.

Note: About a week later we watched the birth video and realized she had been posterior. Just another variation of normal, and definitely not a medical emergency.

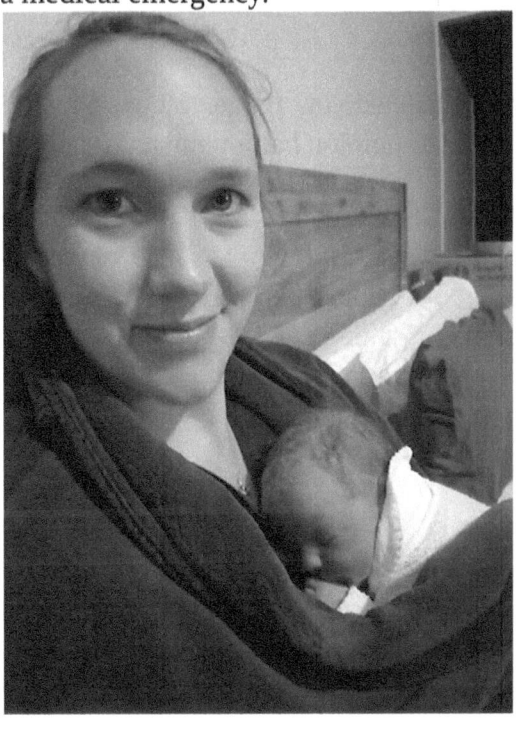

Submit Your Story
And Please Review!

If these stories impacted you, I urge you to go to Amazon.com and review the book! Your opinion has an impact. Please review!

Did these stories inspire you to freebirth, or have you freebirthed before? I'm currently working on a second volume filled with more freebirth stories! If you would like yours to be part of it, please write your story and email it, along with any photos, to:

authorbreemoore@gmail.com

Resources for Your Birth Journey

Books

If there's one thing I do a lot of, it's read! I often joke that I've earned a degree in pregnancy and childbirth with the number of books, studies, websites, etc. that I've read. Here are the ones I recommend most:

- "Unhindered Childbirth: Wisdom for the Passage of Unassisted Birth" by Sarah Morgan Haydock
- "Birth Unhindered: Intimate stories of women experiencing the power and transformation of birth plus a guide to proactive self care" by Tara L. McGuire
- "Unassisted Childbirth" by Laura Kaplan Shanley
- "Home Birth On Your Own Terms: A How To Guide For Birthing Unassisted" by Heather Baker
- "In Search of the Perfect Birth: A Journey From Hospital to Midwife to Unassisted home birth" by Elizabeth X. Rhodes
- "Ina May's Guide to Childbirth" by Ina May Gaskin
- "The Unassisted Baby: A Do-It-Yourself Guide to Pregnancy and Childbirth" by Anita Evensen
- "Unassisted home birth: A Collection of Real Life Stories" by Phyllis Franklin
- "Birthing Freedom: How I Learned to Relax + Have a Baby (After the Nightmare "Natural" Birth of My Firstborn)" by Amanda Grace Harrison
- "Simply Give Birth: A Collection of Stories" by Heather Cushman-Dowdee

- "Supernatural Childbirth" by Jackie Mize
- "Elijah Birth, How to turn the Hearts of the Fathers" by Jenny Hatch
- "Orgasmic Birth: Your Guide to a Safe, Satisfying, and Pleasurable Birth Experience" by Elizabeth Davis and Debra Pascal-Bonaro
- "Mother's Intention: How Belief Shapes Birth" by Kim Wildner and Chelsea Wildner
- "Painless Childbirth: An Empowering Journey Through Pregnancy and Childbirth: An Empowering Journey Through Pregnancy and Birth" by Giuditta Tornetta
- "Birth & Sex: the Power and the Passion" by Sheila Kitzinger

Facebook Groups

Search for the following groups via the Facebook search bar. Follow the instructions carefully when you request to join: many of these groups are strict in who they accept due to internet trolls, etc. This isn't an extensive list. There are dozens of groups out there, but these are the most active, best quality that I can recommend. A warning about Facebook posts: remember that nothing is private on the internet, even in a private group. I hope you find your tribe!

- Unassisted Pregnancy & Childbirth - NO ASSISTANCE TALK
- Unassisted Chilbirth/Freebirth
- Beginners Unassisted Pregnancy & Childbirth Information Group!
- Judgement free UC: Learning about and supporting Unassisted Childbirth
- Transfer stories - Unassisted Childbirth / Freebirth
- Corner Pillar UP/UC - Christian Women
- LDS Unassisted/Freebirth
- Unassisted Birth Doulas

Websites

By no means exhaustive, this list of websites is meant to get you started on your learning path towards freebirth. Here are a few quality sites that have served me well in learning about unassisted pregnancy and childbirth:

- www.unassistedchildbirth.com

- www.freebirthsociety.com - Freebirth Stories, Podcast, and Online Community
- www.indiebirth.org - Freebirth Stories, Podcast, and Resources
- www.birthbecomeshers.weebly.com - Freebirth Stories and Resources
- www.jennyhatch.com - Experienced Unassisted Birther
- www.evidencebasedbirth.com - The BEST studies (for the doubters in your life)
- www.learnbellybinding.com - Learn Postpartum Belly Binding
- Pinterest: Birth Stories and Theories Board by Bree Moore
- Pinterest: Birth Videos for Kids by Bree moore
- www.spinningbabies.com - Learn about optimal positioning for labor and delivery

Podcasts
- The Freebirth Podcast
- Indie Birth Podcast

Films
- Orgasmic Birth: The Best-Kept Secret
- The Business of Being Born
- More Business of Being Born
- Why Not Home
- A Breech in the System
- Laboring Under an Illusion: Mass Media Childbirth vs. the Real Thing

Read More Birth Stories

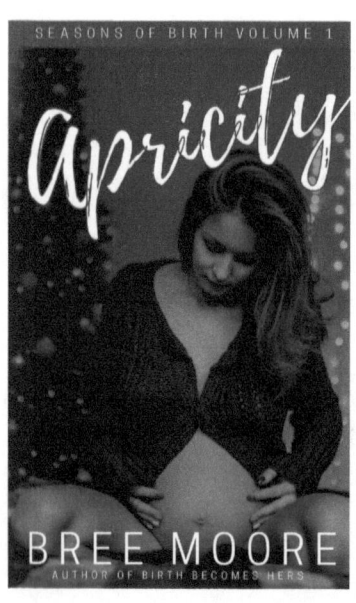

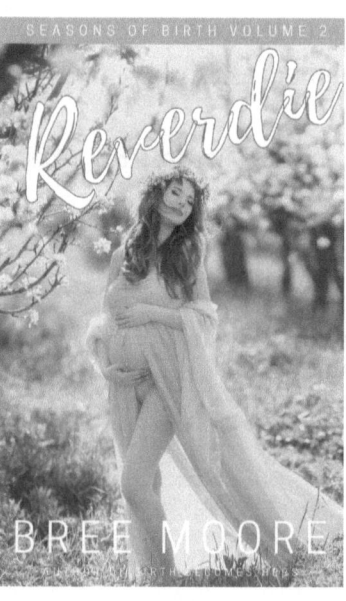

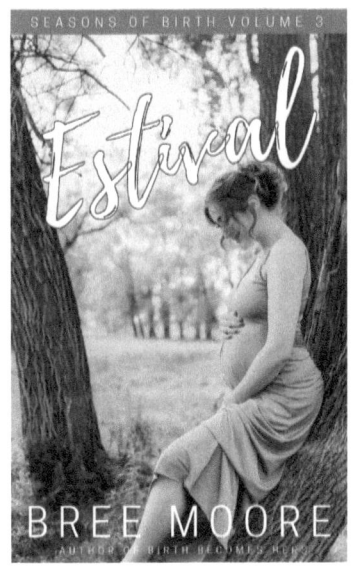
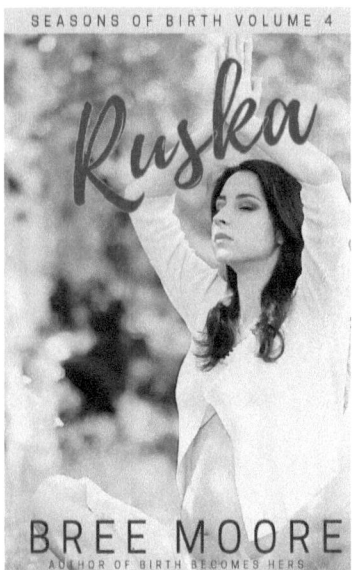

About the Author

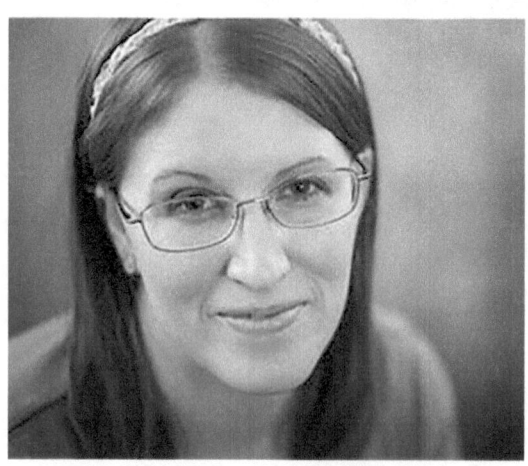

Bree Moore first became involved with birth as a profession after the natural hospital birth of her first child. Her passion grew as she studied childbirth, drawn by the emotional and spiritual implications birth has on the life of both mother and child. She initially trained as a professional postpartum belly binder, helping women recover postpartum, and then later as a birth Doula. She incorporates energy healing into her practice, helping women clear emotional blocks and negative beliefs surrounding pregnancy, birth, and motherhood.

Bree finds great fulfillment in joining women on their journey on the path to motherhood and helping them discover their innate powers of creation through pregnancy and birth. In addition, Bree is a fantasy novelist. She has published numerous novels and short stories. So far all of them contain births! She lives in West Valley

City, Utah, is wife to an amazing "baby-catching" husband and mother to six children, four of which were born at home, unassisted.

http://www.birthbecomeshers.com
https://www.facebook.com/birthbecomeshers
https://www.authorbreemoore.com

Getting Your Spouse or Partner On-board

1 Clarke, Yolande. "Husband or Partner at a Freebirth? Forget Education-Surender & Serve." Bauhauswife, 2018, freebirth.ca/blogs/freebirth/husband-or-partner-at-a-freebirth-forget-education-surender-serve-1.

2 Green, Maryn. "The One About Getting Your Partner 'On Board' With home birth." Indie Birth, 14 Aug. 2015, indiebirth.org/the-one-about-getting-your-partner-on-board-with-home birth/.

3 Harris, Mark. "EVERYTHING You Need to Know When Your Partner Is Pregnant." Birthing4Blokes, 2017, birthing4blokes.com/.

Self-led Pregnancy

1 Green, Maryn. "The Prenatal Supplement Scam: How to Know What You Need." Indie Birth, 6 Mar. 2017, indiebirth.org/prenatal-supplement-scam-know-need/.

2 Shanley, Laura Kaplan. "Eating During Pregnancy: Indulge Yourself." Unassisted Childbirth, www.unassistedchildbirth.com/inspiration/eating-during-pregnancy-indulge-yourself/.

"Natural" Induction Methods

1 Dekker, Rebecca. "The Evidence on: Due Dates." Evidence Based Birth®, 26 Feb. 2019, evidencebasedbirth.com/evidence-on-inducing-labor-for-going-past-your-due-date/.

Placentas and Post-birth Bleeding

1 Green, Maryn. "Exposing the Postpartum Hemorrhage Deception." Indie Birth, 30 Apr. 2014, www.indiebirth.org/exposing-the-postpartum-hemorrhage-deception/?fbclid=IwAR3x15Wlkg8_MsrCcARRZGcNqMpHgWm-wAJqFBaDYPVv1ms1xn9zDW593VM.

What if I Tear?

1 Gilpin-Blake , Denise, and Summer Elliott. "A Natural Alternative to Suturing." Midwifery Today, 10 Apr. 2018, midwiferytoday.com/mt-articles/natural-alternative-suturing/.

The Wisdom found in Not-Knowing

1 Clarke, Yolande. "Unpacking Ultrasound With Yolande Clark." SoundCloud, Apr. 2018, soundcloud.com/user-754199824/unpacking-ultrasound-with-yolande-clarke.

Finding Intuition
1 Google Search Dictionary, search result for "Define Intuition"

www.ingramcontent.com/pod-product-compliance
Lightning Source LLC
Chambersburg PA
CBHW020755230426
43673CB00022B/443/J